Introducing, Designing *and* Conducting Research *for* **Paramedics**

Introducing, Designing *and* Conducting Research *for* Paramedics

EDITORS

ALEXANDER OLAUSSEN BEmergHlth(Paramedic), BMedSc(Hons),
MBBS(Hons), MACPara, FHEA
Department of Paramedicine
Monash University, Australia;
National Trauma Research Institute, The Alfred, Australia;
Centre for Research and Evaluation, Ambulance Victoria, Australia

KELLY-ANN BOWLES BSc(Human Movement Sc),
GradDipBiostats, PhD
Department of Paramedicine
School of Primary and Allied Healthcare
Monash University, Australia

BILL LORD BHlthSc(PreHospCare), GradDipCBL, MEd, PhD
Department of Paramedicine
Monash University, Australia

BRETT WILLIAMS BAVEd, BHlthSc, Grad Cert IntensiveCareParamedicine,
Grad Dip EmergHlth, MHlthSc, PhD, FACP
Department of Paramedicine
Monash University, Australia

ELSEVIER

ELSEVIER

Elsevier Australia. ACN 001 002 357
(a division of Reed International Books Australia Pty Ltd)
Tower 1, 475 Victoria Avenue, Chatswood, NSW 2067

ISBN: 978-0-7295-4409-2

Notice

Practitioners and researchers must always rely on their own experience and knowledge in evaluating and using any information, methods, compounds or experiments described herein. Because of rapid advances in the medical sciences, in particular, independent verification of diagnoses and drug dosages should be made. To the fullest extent of the law, no responsibility is assumed by Elsevier, authors, editors or contributors for any injury and/or damage to persons or property as a matter of products liability, negligence or otherwise, or from any use or operation of any methods, products, instructions, or ideas contained in the material herein.

National Library of Australia Cataloguing-in-Publication Data

 A catalogue record for this book is available from the National Library of Australia

Content Strategist: Elizabeth Ryan
Content Project Manager: Shubham Dixit
Edited by Leanne Peters
Proofread by Melissa Faulkner
Permissions Editing and Photo Research: Regina Lavanya Remigius
Cover design by Gopalakrishnan Venkatraman
Index by Innodata
Typeset by GW India
Printed in Singapore by KHL Printing Co Pte Ltd

Last digit is the print number: 9 8 7 6 5 4 3 2 1

CONTENTS

SECTION 3 Explaining the What (Quantitative)

SECTION 4 Explaining the Why (Qualitative)

SECTION 5 Other Ways to Answer the Question

SECTION 6 Sharing New Knowledge

PART TEN   Disseminating and Implementing Research

PART ELEVEN   The Future of Paramedicine Research, Summary and Conclusion

PREFACE

Paramedicine is an established profession in some countries, and an emerging profession in others. Entry-to-practice education is increasingly university-based, and the amount of discipline-specific evidence underpinning paramedicine is rapidly expanding, with a unique classification for paramedicine research recently approved in Australia and New Zealand. Other jurisdictions like United Kingdom are also following suit when it comes to the true acknowledgment of paramedicine as its own area of research, and this vital step will, without a doubt, have positive international implications.

A cornerstone underpinning a profession is having its own unique body of knowledge or theory. A critical step in building a body of knowledge is generating and publishing high-quality scientific work in peer-reviewed journals. This research typically arises from the identification of clinical, operational or professional questions that need to be answered in order to inform practice and policy.

A recent review completed by some of the editors of this book found that that only 12% of the top 100 most-cited articles relating to paramedicine were led by paramedics. This is a lost opportunity, because not only are paramedics the eyes and ears directly experiencing issues that need improvement or further investigation to understand the problem (and thus research by extension), they are also the heads and hands that will be implementing the new evidence. However, paramedics have traditionally had less opportunities to lead research when compared to other health and medical professionals. This lack of research confidence and 'know-how' are the first barriers we need to overcome in the development of a strong paramedic research community.

The aim of this book is to introduce paramedics and out-of-hospital clinicians to the principles and practice of research, in the hope it will support understanding of the importance of scientific enquiry, educate paramedics about the importance of research and evidence-based practice, and inspire paramedics to undertake research or even consider research as a career opportunity.

A unique textbook for research in paramedicine – compared to the many generic resources that exist – is required because many of the core concepts in research have special challenges when carried out in the paramedic practice setting. We also believe that a dedicated book like this will be more engaging and assist your learning and understanding through the use of real-life out-of-hospital topics and trials.

There is more to paramedicine than, for instance, deciding on whether or not epinephrine is indicated in cardiac arrest. Equally important topics include the wellbeing and education of paramedics, as well as expanding the role of paramedic-led healthcare. All these topics require different research approaches, which is why we have covered several methodologies in this book.

We have split this book up into more than 50 chapters to function as a rapid-reference manual. We have deliberately kept the chapters succinct to enhance the conceptual understanding, avoiding details that may be unnecessarily complex. Each chapter is instead supplemented by a list of further readings and suggested resources for the reader to explore in further detail. So, in short, this book should serve as the first step in your research journey.

SUGGESTED AUDIENCE

The primary audience of this book is the paramedic or out-of-hospital clinician who is looking to start their research journey or expand their current research knowledge. As the area of paramedicine research is developing, we are finding more paramedics and out-of-hospital clinicians are broadening their education and developing their own research skills. This may be occurring in structured academic courses, or may be through a self-directed expansion to one's own knowledge. Regardless of the approach to this new skill development, the pathway into research can be very daunting. With so much information available, it can be difficult for a new researcher to know where to start. This book is designed with that trepidation and confusion in mind. There is no presumption of knowledge before you open it. For some, this book may reinforce some of their current knowledge, while expanding their horizons to other research approaches. Either way, this book should offer every reader the opportunity to gain a basic understanding of the diverse aspects of research.

ACKNOWLEDGMENTS

Paramedicine research is well known for its networks and collaborative approach. The development of this book is no different. As can be seen by reviewing the contributor's names and locations, this book represents the four corners of the globe, showing the diverse and expansive skill set of paramedicine researchers internationally. These people have given their time and expertise for the development of the next generation of paramedicine researchers. All have contributed to this book because they understand the exciting time that paramedicine research is currently in, and they hope that their contribution will help develop research passion in paramedics for years to come.

We hope that you will find this resource useful and look forward to reading your completed research in print. Your contribution to the body of paramedicine evidence will not only help patients and paramedics in all pertinent areas, but also leave a legacy of a foundational stone in the evolution of paramedicine.

CONTRIBUTORS

Talal AlShammari PhD
Department of Emergency Medical Care, College of Applied
   Medical Sciences, Imam Abdulrahman bin Faisal
   University, Saudi Arabia

Ibrahim Althagafi BParamedic,
   MSci(DisasterMedManagement), PhD candidate
College of Health and Medicine, School of Nursing,
   University of Tasmania, Australia

Natalie Elizabeth Anderson RN, BA, BHSc,
   MSc(Hons), PhD
Faculty of Medical and Health Sciences, University
   of Auckland, New Zealand;
Auckland City Hospital Emergency Department,
   New Zealand

Emily Andrew BSc(Biomedical), MBiostat,
   PhD candidate
Department of Epidemiology and Preventive Medicine,
   Monash University, Australia;
Centre for Research and Evaluation, Ambulance Victoria,
   Australia

Richard Armour BParamedPrac, MSc,
   MParamedicine(CriticalCare)
Ambulance Victoria Australia;
Monash University, Australia

Leon Baranowski MSc(AdvPract), MEd(ClinEd)
British Columbia Emergency Health Services, Canada;
Justice Institute of British Columbia, Canada

Alan M Batt PGCME, MSc, PhD, FHEA
Department of Paramedicine, Monash University, Australia;
Paramedic Programs, Fanshawe College, Canada

Bronwyn Beovich BAppSc, MChSc
Department of Paramedicine, Monash University, Australia

Audrey L Blewer MPH, PhD
Department of Family Medicine and Community Health,
   Department of Population Health Sciences,
   Duke University School of Medicine, United States;
Department of Health Services and Systems Research,
   Duke-NUS Medical School, Singapore

Ted Brown BScOT(Hons), GCHPE, OT(C), OTR,
   MRCOT, MSc, MPA, PhD, FOTARA, FAOTA
Department of Occupational Therapy, School of Primary
   and Allied Health Care, Faculty of Medicine, Nursing
   and Health Sciences, Monash University, Australia

Madison Brydges MA, PhD candidate
Department of Health Aging & Society, McMaster University,
   Hamilton, Canada

Yu-Tung Chang PhD(HealthPromotion&HealthEd)
Taiwan Society of Paramedicine, Taiwan

Niamh M Cummins BSc, MSc, PhD
School of Medicine, University of Limerick, Ireland;
Irish Paramedicine Education and Research Network
   (IPERN), Ireland

Tom Davidson MCPara, BSc(Hons), MSc, PhD
   candidate, HEA fellow
Centre of Excellence in Paramedic Practice, Institute of
   Health, University of Cumbria, United Kingdom

Dale G Edwards BHlthSci(Paramedic),
   GradCertEd(Workplace Training and Assessment),
   Med(Curriculum Design), EdD, FACPara
Paramedicine Program, Tasmanian School of Medicine,
   University of Tasmania, Australia

Belinda Flanagan AssocDipSci(Ambulance),
   BApplSci(Nurs), GradCertProfLearning, MPH,
   Mid, PhD
Tasmanian School of Medicine, University
   of Tasmania, Australia

Jonathan Foo BPhysio(Hons), PhD
Department of Physiotherapy, School of Primary and Allied
   Health Care, Faculty of Medicine, Nursing and Health
   Sciences, Monash University, Australia;
Society for Cost and Value in Health Professions Education,
   Australia

Susan Furness BEmergHlth(Paramedic), PhD
Department Rural Community Health, La Trobe Rural
   Health School, Australia

Cameron McRae Gosling BAppSc(HM),
Grad Dip(Ex Rehab), MAppSc(Research), PhD
Department of Paramedicine, Monash University, Australia

Jennie S Helmer Advanced Care Paramedic, MEd
School of Population and Public Health, University of British
Columbia, Canada;
Paramedic Academy, Justice Institute of British Columbia,
Canada;
British Columbia Emergency Health Services, Canada

Andrew Fu Wah Ho MBBS, MMED, MPH
Department of Emergency Medicine, Singapore General
Hospital, Singapore;
Pre-hospital and Emergency Research Center, Duke-NUS
Medical School, Singapore

Gemma Howlett BSc(Hons), MSc, MCPara,
PhD candidate, HEA Senior Fellow
University of Cumbria, United Kingdom

Ross Anthony Iles BPhysio(Hons),
GradDipWorkDisabilityPrevention, PhD
School of Public Health and Preventive Medicine,
Monash University, Australia

Paul Andrew Jennings BNur, GradCertAdvNsg,
GradCertBiostats, GCHPE, MClinEpi, PhD
Ambulance Victoria, Australia;
Department of Paramedicine and Department of
Epidemiology and Preventive Medicine, Monash
University, Australia

Liam Langford BHSci(Paramedic), GradCertHEd,
MPublicHealth
Australasian College of Paramedicine, Australia

William J Leggio, Jr NRP, EdD
Office of the Chief Medical Officer, Austin/Travis County
EMS System and City of Austin, United States

Nan Liu PhD
Centre for Quantitative Medicine and Programme, Health
Services and Systems Research (HSSR), Duke-NUS
Medical School, Singapore

David Nicholas Long AdvDip ParaSc,
BHlthSc(Pre-HospCare), BEd(Hab),
GradCertAcadPrac, PhD, FHEA
Paramedic Science, School of Health and Medical Sciences,
University of Southern Queensland, Australia

Stephen Maloney BPhysio, MPH, MBA, PhD
Department of Physiotherapy, School of Primary and Allied
Health Care, Faculty of Medicine, Nursing and Health
Sciences, Monash University, Australia;
Society for Cost and Value in Health Professions Education,
Australia

Ong Eng Hock Marcus MBBS, MPH, FRCS
Department of Emergency Medicine, Singapore General
Hospital, Singapore;
Health Services and Systems Research (HSSR), Duke-NUS
Medical School, Singapore

Ben Meadley DipParamedSci, BAppSci,
GradCertAeromed, GradDipEmerg Health,
GradDipIntensiveCareParamed, PhD, FACPara
Department of Paramedicine, Monash University, Australia;
Ambulance Victoria, Australia

Navindhra (Navin) Naidoo NDip(AEC), HDipEd,
BTech(EMC), MPH, PhD (Forensic Medicine)
School of Health Sciences, Western Sydney University,
Australia;
Australasian College of Paramedicine, Australia

Koshi Nakagawa MEM, EMT-P
Graduate School of Emergency Medical System, Kokushikan
University, Japan

Ziad Nehme BEmergHlth(Paramedic)(Hons), PhD,
ASM, FACPara
Department of Epidemiology and Preventive Medicine,
and Department of Paramedicine, Monash University,
Australia;
Centre for Research and Evaluation, Ambulance Victoria,
Australia

Yilin Ning PhD
Centre for Quantitative Medicine (CQM), Duke-NUS
Medical School, United States

Peter Francis O'Meara BHA, GradCertAgHlthMed,
MPP, PhD
Department of Paramedicine, Monash University, Australia;
The Paramedic Network, Australia

Gerard M O'Reilly MBBS, MPH, MBiostat, AStat,
PhD, FACEM
School of Public Health and Preventive Medicine, Monash
University, Australia;
Emergency and Trauma Centre, The Alfred, Australia;
National Trauma Research Institute, The Alfred, Australia

Alaa O Oteir PhD
Department of Allied Medical Sciences, Faculty of Applied
    Medical Sciences, Jordan University of Science
    and Technology, Jordan;
Department of Paramedicine, Monash University, Australia

**Robin Pap BTechEMC, NDipEMC, HDipHET,
    MScMed(EmergMed)**
Western Sydney University, Australia

Douglas Paton PhD
College of Health and Human Sciences, Charles Darwin
    University, Australia

Nigel Rees BSc(Hons), MSc, QAM, PhD, FCpara
Welsh Ambulance Service NHS Trust, Wales

**David Reid DipHlthSci, BSci(Paramedical Science),
    GradCert HSM, GAICD, MHM(Hons),
    MACPara, PhD**
School of Medical and Health Sciences, Edith Cowan
    University, Australia

Louise Reynolds BHSc, MPH, PGCertHE, PhD, FACP
Victoria University, Australia

Luke Robinson BOccTherapy(Hons), PhD, FHEA
Department of Occupational Therapy, School of Primary and
    Allied Health Care, Faculty of Medicine, Nursing
    and Health Sciences, Monash University, Australia

Ryo Sagisaka PhD, EMT-P
Department of Integrated Science and Engineering
    for Sustainable Societies, Chuo University, Japan;
Research Institute of Disaster Management and EMS,
    Kokushikan University, Japan

**Brendan Shannon BEmergHealth(PMed)(Hons),
    PhD candidate**
Department of Paramedicine, Monash University, Australia

**Paul Simpson AdvDipParamedScience(ICP),
    BHSc(PrehospCare), BEd(PD/H/PE),
    GradCert(PaedEmerg), GradCert(ClinEd),
    MScM(ClinEpi), PhD**
Western Sydney University, Australia

**Erin Claire SmithBhlthInfoManagement, MPH,
    MClinEpi, PhD**
Dentistry and Health Sciences, Faculty of Medicine,
    Melbourne University, Australia

Karen Smith BSc, PhD
Centre for Research and Evaluation, Ambulance Victoria,
    Australia;
Department of Epidemiology and Preventive Medicine,
    Department of Paramedicine, Monash University,
    Australia

**Lindsay Mervyn Smith RN, BHlthSci, GradCertUniL&T,
    MNS, PhD**
School of Nursing, University of Tasmania, Australia

Hideharu Tanaka MD, PhD
Graduate School of Emergency Medical System, Research
    Institute of Disaster Management and EMS, Kokushikan
    University, Department of Sports Medicine, Kokushikan
    University, Japan

Shota Tanaka BS, ATC, EMT-P
Research Institute of Disaster Management and EMS,
    Kokushikan University, Japan

Walter Tavares ACP, PhD
Department of Paramedicine, Monash University, Australia;
The Wilson Centre and Temerty Faculty of Medicine,
    University Health Network, University of Toronto,
    Canada;
Institute of Health Policy, Management and Evaluation
    (IHPME), Dalla Lana School of Public Health, University
    of Toronto, Canada;
York Region Paramedic and Senior Services, Community
    Health Services Department, Regional Municipality of
    York, Canada

Kieran Walsh MB, FRCPI
BMJ Learning and Quality, BMJ, London, United Kingdom;
Society for Cost and Value in Health Professions Education,
    Australia

**Sam Willis BSc(ParamedicSci)(Hons), MAEd(research),
    PhD candidate**
Curtin University, Australia

You You PhD
Institute of Economics of Education and Institute of Medical
    Education, Peking University, China;
Society for Cost and Value in Health Professions Education,
    Australia

SECTION 1

Introduction to Research

This book is divided into six different sections. First, the reader is introduced to research from a historical and professional point of view (Section 1). We then detail how to prepare for the research experience (Section 2) and how to conduct quantitative (Section 3) and qualitative (Section 4) research. Other research methodologies are discussed in Section 5. Finally, we discuss how to disseminate and share your research (Section 6).

In this first section, we first present research within healthcare from a historical perspective (Chapter 1), why research is important for the paramedic profession (Chapter 2) and what evidence-based practice within paramedicine looks like (Chapter 3). Before launching into the specifics of research, we outline some thoughts on how to use this book (Chapter 4).

The second half of this first section (Part Two) is called 'Starting at the start'. How to determine what to research is often the first hurdle for many students, and this is addressed in Chapter 5. We then discuss how to design a well-formulated question (Chapter 6) as well as tips on what to do before commencing your research (Chapter 7). The reader is then introduced to key frameworks (Chapter 8) and where in the evidence hierarchy different pieces of research—including your own—fit (Chapter 9). A discussion of ethics (Chapter 10) then concludes this first section.

1

Historical Perspectives and the Emergence of Research in Healthcare

Talal AlShammari

LEARNING OUTCOMES

1. Understand the basic timeline in the historical development of research in healthcare
2. Recognise the contributions of historical figures associated with research in healthcare
3. Outline the historical phases in the development of clinical trials

INTRODUCTION

The search for knowledge in healthcare has a long and varied tradition across different cultures. This can be seen from the view of maintenance of personal health, such as the need to identify plants of healing or poisonous properties. The earliest known evidence of healthcare can be attributed to the Ebers Papyrus from ancient Egypt, which contains important medical papyri dating back to 1550 BCE.[1] The library of Ashurbanipal from Mesopotamia was also an important source of ancient clay tablets describing mineral and vegetable drugs.[2,3] In addition, the Pen-ts'ao Ching, attributed to the ancient mythological Chinese emperor Shen Nung, contains more than 100 medicinal plants.[2]

All human cultures developed their own form of healthcare practice, whether written or passed on from generation to generation. However, developing knowledge based on an empirical understanding is a product of the scientific method. Historically, the early rudimentary rise of the scientific method has been attributed to Ancient Greece.[4,5] This tradition was then carried on through a long period of translation and development, with some scholarly works translated into Arabic.[4] Finally, the scientific method went through an accelerated phase of development in the Renaissance and Enlightenment periods up to our modern times.[6] This chapter aims to provide an account of the emergence of healthcare research and its applicability following the development of the scientific method.

MILESTONES IN THE EMERGENCE OF RESEARCH IN HEALTHCARE

Controlled Clinical Trials

The development of healthcare research was empirically established in the 18th century, with the first modern controlled clinical trial by James Lind in 1747, for the treatment of scurvy.[7] The second phase in the development of clinical trials was the use of a placebo as a control to the treatment group. This was done by Austin Flint in 1863, for the treatment of rheumatism.[8] The final major historical development was the concurrent introduction of a double-blind controlled trial in 1943 and randomised curative trials in 1946, for the common cold and pulmonary tuberculosis, respectively.[8] While many research designs are available to healthcare providers, randomised controlled trials are still generally considered to be the gold standard in identifying causality, which continues to be the primary aim of research since ancient times.

Evolution Of Vaccine Development

The introduction of vaccines is one of the most significant scientific contributions to human health. A great example can be seen in the story of smallpox, where a highly contagious disease with a 30% mortality rate was widespread throughout the world.[9-11] In 1796, Edward Jenner tested the common myth that milkmaidens who got cowpox were not affected by smallpox. The experiment was undertaken by inoculating a young James Phipps with cowpox. Mr. Phipps was then exposed to smallpox and was found to be immune to the disease. Although, the ethics of Dr. Jenner's research may be unacceptable to our modern research practice, he went on to publish his findings in 1798.[12] The ultimate result of Edward Jenner's experiment was the eradication of the smallpox disease by 1980, through widespread vaccination campaigns.[10]

The Antibiotic Age

In 1928, Alexander Fleming walked into his lab after a holiday respite and found one of his samples had been contaminated.[13] After experimentation, he published the following in the *British Journal of Experimental Pathology*: 'It was found that broth in which the mould had been grown at room temperature for one or two weeks had acquired marked inhibitory, bactericidal and bacteriolytic properties to many of the more common pathogenic bacteria'.[14] Although he did not realise it at the time, Sir Alexander had introduced the world to the antibiotic age. These drugs would go on to alter human health in such a radical way that they became a principal reason for the removal of communicable diseases from being the leading cause of death in Western countries.[9]

As can be seen from the previous examples diseases can be eradicated, or their effect lessened, by using drugs or vaccines. In our current times, the world is collectively able to tackle the COVID-19 pandemic using drugs and vaccines that are empirically tested using controlled clinical trials. Thus, health research was and will continue to be the doctrine for evidence-based practice.

CONCLUSION

The desire to know more is a genuine aspect of human nature. From the primal times of our existence we have observed, experimented and discovered the true nature of our world. Yet our ancient methods have always been either subjective or unrecorded, until the birth of the scientific method. From that time, the theoretical concept of the scientific method has been translated to the benefit of

human health with different research designs, especially through the gold standard of controlled clinical trials. This chapter has produced an account of the historical rise of healthcare research and its contribution to human health.

REVIEW QUESTIONS

1. In your opinion, what is the most important research contribution to human health?
2. How can paramedics integrate health research into their profession?
3. Should health research be part of a paramedic's continuous education practice? Explain your answer.

SUGGESTED FURTHER READING

Kumar R. Research methodology: a step-by-step guide for beginners. 5th ed. London: SAGE; 2018.

REFERENCES

1. Marte A, Caldamone AA, Aguir LM. The history of the pediatric inguinal hernia repair. Journal of Pediatric Urology. 2021;17(4):485–91.
2. Janick J. Herbals: the connection between horticulture and medicine. HortTechnology. 2003;13(2):229. Online. Available: http://doi.org/10.21273/horttech.13.2.0229.
3. Retief F, Cilliers L. Mesopotamian medicine. South African Medical Journal. 2007;97(1):27–30.
4. De Lacy OL. How Greek science passed to the Arabs. Cumbernuld: Ares Publishers; 1949.
5. Kattsoff LO. Ptolemy and scientific method: a note on the history of an idea. Isis. 1947;38(1/2):18–22.
6. Gower B. Scientific method: a historical and philosophical introduction. Abingdon: Taylor and Francis; 1997.
7. Collier R. Legumes, lemons and streptomycin: a short history of the clinical trial. Canadian Medical Association Journal. 2009;180(1):23–4. Online. Available: http://doi.org/10.1503/cmaj.081879.
8. Bhatt A. Evolution of clinical research: a history before and beyond James Lind. Perspectives in Clinical Research. 2010;1(1):6.
9. Adedeji WA. The treasure called antibiotics. Annals of Ibadan Postgraduate Medicine. 2016;14(2):56–7. Online. Available: https://pubmed.ncbi.nlm.nih.gov/28337088.
10. Breman JG, Henderson DA. Diagnosis and management of smallpox. New England Journal of Medicine. 2002;346(17):1300–8. Online. Available: http://doi.org/10.1056/NEJMra020025.
11. MacIntyre CR, Costantino V, Chen X, Segelov E, Chughtai, AA, Kelleher A, et al. Influence of population immunosuppression and past vaccination on smallpox reemergence. Emerging Infectious Disease Journal. 2018;24(4):646. Online. Available: http://doi.org/10.3201/eid2404.171233.

12. Stewart AJ, Devlin PM. The history of the smallpox vaccine. Journal of Infection. 2006;52(5):329–34. Online. Available: http://doi.org/10.1016/j.jinf.2005.07.021.

13. Tan SY, Tatsumura Y. Alexander Fleming (1881–1955): discoverer of penicillin. Singapore Medical Journal. 2015;56(7):366–7. Online. Available: http://doi.org/10.11622/smedj.2015105.

14. Fleming A. On the antibacterial action of cultures of a Penicillium, with special reference to their use in the isolation of B. influenzæ. British Journal of Experimental Pathology. 1929;10(3):226–36. Online. Available: https://www.ncbi.nlm.nih.gov/pmc/articles/PMC2048009/.

The Importance of Research for Paramedicine as a Profession

William J Leggio and Niamh M Cummins

LEARNING OUTCOMES

1. Identify professional aspects of paramedicine influenced by research
2. Describe the intersections of research and the paramedicine profession
3. Demonstrate an understanding of the importance of research for paramedicine as a profession

INTRODUCTION

The publication of this book focused on research for paramedicine, authored by leading international researchers, likely serves as a pinnacle for our profession across developed and developing countries. Research remains a professional gap in paramedicine regardless of the level of sophistication of the system or level of practice. There are examples of completed national emergency medical services (EMS) research agendas aimed to influence the profession by highlighting research gaps and opportunities to better understand the profession and patient care.[1–5] There are similar examples advocating for international[6] or national research agendas,[7] and strategies related to research[8] or evidence-based guidelines[9].

Historically, paramedicine has relied on 'heirloom knowledge' or on evidence generated by other health professions. Though there are certainly a few notable exceptions, paramedicine researchers remain a small but growing community. Paramedicine researchers are producing peer-reviewed scholarly contributions; however, many EMS and out-of-hospital publications are frequently still led or completely authored by non-paramedic clinicians such as physicians or nurses.[10]

One way for the profession to grow autonomy beyond that enjoyed when providing out-of-hospital patient care is by leading original research. Through research, the profession can evaluate evidence and determine practice decisions rather than relying on researchers from different clinical disciplines to lead such efforts. This is not to dismiss the importance of collaboration and interprofessional approaches to conducting research as paramedicine itself serves many functions between medicine, public safety and public health. The growth and appreciation for research in paramedicine that culminated in the publication of this book hopefully represents a critical mass for the profession to demonstrate a basis and value for its practice, clinician education and performance of service providers.

The following are examples of the broad-ranging impact of a research-rich environment on key aspects of the paramedic profession.

RESEARCH-INFORMED PRACTICE AND PATIENT OUTCOMES IN PARAMEDICINE

Research-informed practice is a key component of modern healthcare, and health services benefit from research through an overall improvement in the quality of patient care and increased patient safety. Demonstrating improved quality of patient care requires research using patient outcome data and development of evidence-based practice (EBP). Although discussed more in Chapter 3, a strong research culture is vital in EBP; however, this has developed more slowly in paramedicine. Providers broadly document the response to out-of-hospital interventions, but the concept of researching the quality of patient care and patient outcomes does extend beyond out-of-hospital data. The continuum of care the patient receives during the same encounter is also vitally important. This separation in research may be attributed to the fact that research is more challenging in the out-of-hospital setting; however, paramedicine is both dynamic and innovative and is rapidly evolving.

RESEARCH AND CLINICIAN EDUCATION IN THE PARAMEDIC PROFESSION

Traditionally, education in paramedicine had been vocational 'on the road' training which meant there had been less focus on research and evaluation skills. Internationally, many jurisdictions have progressed to a higher education model and research literacy has developed significantly in paramedicine. However, to be recognised as healthcare professionals on an equal footing with nursing, medicine and other allied health professions it is necessary for paramedics and learners to become more than just research consumers. This likely requires a deepened education pedagogy for both initial and continued education strategies related to research-informed practice and research competencies. In order to bridge the evidence-practice gap, paramedicine as a profession needs to focus on knowledge generation, knowledge translation and evidence implementation.

RESEARCH, PROFESSIONALISATION AND THE PERFORMANCE OF SERVICE PROVIDERS

Fostering a learning culture is foundational for service providers to support the role of research in the paramedicine profession. Just as clinicians have a role in being more than research consumers, so do service providers. This includes researching best practices in retaining staff, increased job satisfaction and workforce safety as just a few examples. Service providers also have roles in researching the translation of both clinical and operational evidence into practice and they also need to support, mentor and cultivate paramedicine researchers. Accountability to outcomes and implementation of clinical and operational evidence likely requires service providers to support quality assurance and performance improvement activities. Quality assurance research is one function service providers have in assessing consistency of care and quality of clinical decisions, as two examples. Systems thinking and performance improvement provide service providers with frameworks and approaches to improve variance and processes influencing clinical and operational outcomes.

CONCLUSION

The importance of research and knowledge translation for paramedicine as a profession cannot be understated. Key reasons for building research capacity in the paramedic profession include improving outcomes for patients, enhancing job satisfaction and confidence for clinicians, and optimising performance, efficiency and staff retention for EMS providers. There is a need for increased research in the profession and particularly for research which is paramedic driven and led. This will enable paramedics to evolve beyond being research consumers through becoming research generators and research implementers of their own profession. This may require an evolution of roles in the profession and particularly a clearly defined career pathway for researchers in paramedicine. To bridge the evidence-practice gap will require multiple methodological approaches and expertise in observational and experimental research methods including collection and analysis of quantitative and qualitative data. This chapter has just highlighted broad reasons for the importance of increasing paramedicine research rather than attempting to craft an exhaustive list. Reading this book and published EMS literature will provide insights to the totality of the gaps in our professional body of research. In terms of professionalisation, paramedics can become masters of their own destiny, and research is key to achieving this goal.

REVIEW QUESTIONS

1. What are your thoughts on shifting the paramedicine profession from research consumers to generators and implementers?
2. What strengths and weaknesses do paramedics have that will facilitate the building of research capacity within the profession?
3. In your opinion, what research topics should be prioritised for paramedicine as a profession?

SUGGESTED FURTHER READING

The National EMS Research Agenda Writing Team. National EMS Research Agenda [Internet]. National Highway Traffic Safety Administration; 2001 Dec. Report No.: DTN 22-99-H-05100. Online. Available: https://www.ems.gov/pdf/National_EMS_Research_Agenda_2001.pdf

Martin-Gill C, Gaither JB, Bigham BL, Myers JB, Kupas DF, Spaite DW. National Prehospital Evidence-Based Guidelines Strategy: A Summary for EMS Stakeholders. Prehosp Emerg Care. 2016 Mar 3;20(2):175–83.

REFERENCES

1. The National EMS Research Agenda Writing Team. National EMS Research Agenda. Prehospital Emergency Care. 2002 Jan;6(sup3):1–43.

2. van de Glind I, Berben S, Zeegers F, Poppen H, Hoogeveen M, Bolt I, et al. A national research agenda for pre-hospital emergency medical services in the Netherlands: a Delphi-study. Scandinavian Journal of Trauma, Resuscitation and Emergency. 2016 Dec;24(1):2.

3. Jensen JL, Bigham BL, Blanchard IE, Dainty KN, Socha D, Carter A, et al. The Canadian National EMS Research Agenda: a mixed methods consensus study. Canadian Journal of Emergency Medicine. 2013 Mar;15(02):73–82.

4. O'Donnel C, O'Reilly S. A National Prehospital Research Strategy. Limerick, Ireland: Centre for Prehospital Research University of Limerick; 2008.

5. The National EMS Research Agenda Writing Team. National EMS Research Agenda. National Highway Traffic Safety Administration; 2001 Dec. Report No.: DTN 22-99-H-05100. Online. Available: https://www.ems.gov/pdf/National_EMS_Research_Agenda_2001.pdf.

6. Maguire B, O'Meara P, Newton A. Toward an international paramedic research agenda. Irish Journal of Paramedicine. 2016;1(2).

7. O'Meara P, Maguire B, Jennings P, Simpson P. Building an Australasian paramedicine research agenda: a narrative review. Health Research Policy and Systems. 2015 Dec;13(1):79.

8. Sayre MR, White LJ, Brown LH, McHenry SD. The National EMS Research Strategic Plan. Prehospital Emergency Care. 2005 Jan;9(3):255–66.

9. Martin-Gill C, Gaither JB, Bigham BL, Myers JB, Kupas DF, Spaite DW. National Prehospital Evidence-Based Guidelines Strategy: A Summary for EMS Stakeholders. Prehospital Emergency Care. 2016 Mar 3;20(2):175–83.

10. Beovich B, Olaussen A, Williams B. A bibliometric analysis of paramedicine publications using Scopus database: 2010–2019. International Emergency Nursing. 2021 Nov, 59:101077.

Evidence-Based Practice for Paramedicine

Kelly-Ann Bowles

LEARNING OUTCOMES

1. Understand the evidence-based medicine triad
2. Understand the steps involved in evidence-based practice implementation
3. Apply the concept of evidence-based practice to the paramedicine field

INTRODUCTION

A paramedic attending a patient considers a number of factors before they commence their clinical treatment. They talk to their patient to find out what led to the emergency call; they consider the clinical practice guidelines of their service; and they use their own clinical judgment. Without even labelling it, the paramedic has used the evidence-based medicine triad, combining the three components of the patient, the research and their own expertise equally, to inform their clinical decision-making. By doing so they aim to provide optimal care for their patient, while treating the patient as a person with their own individual circumstances.

In the 1990s, Sackett and colleagues defined the area of evidence-based medicine as 'the conscientious, explicit and judicious use of current best evidence in making decisions about the care of individual patients'.[1] However, research alone cannot determine the best treatment for a patient. As clinicians internationally would agree, a treatment for a medical condition may work very well for one patient and fail miserably for another. Therefore, evidence-based practice expands on the evidence-based medicine principle, ensuring that the clinician not only uses the latest evidence in determining treatment, they also consider the values, circumstances and preferences of the patient, as well as their own clinical experience. This concept may be even more important in paramedic practice settings, where current research evidence may primarily be completed in the hospital settings. The

paramedic clinician then needs to incorporate their own clinical expertise and patient's circumstances when deciding on the treatment approach. When it comes to research evidence, most paramedics would rely on their service's clinical practice guidelines reinforced by the Australian National Health and Medical Research Council statement that 'clinical practice guidelines are evidence-based statements that include recommendations intended to optimise patient care and assist healthcare practitioners to make decisions about appropriate healthcare for specific clinical circumstances'.[2]

Formalising paramedic education and training and improving community health literacy will enhance two components of the evidence-based practice model. However, increasing the quality and diversity of paramedic-specific research is vital to complete the evidence-based practice triad. Likewise, no paramedic or paramedicine researcher has the time to read all research, and therefore must rely on consortiums and ambulance services to ensure that their clinical practice guidelines are based on the best quality and jurisdiction relevant evidence.

In addition to describing the evidence-based practice triad, Sackett and colleagues established a five-step framework to guide the implementation of research findings.[1] They believed that the framework should be viewed as a cycle, as the results would encourage further research development to continue to improve patient care. As can be seen in Figure 3.1, the initial five steps of the evidence-based practice framework focused on the 5 As of *ask*,

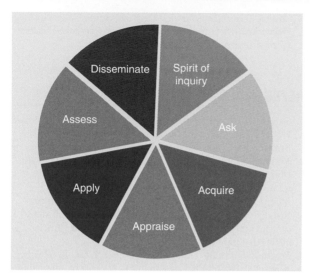

Figure 3.1 The seven steps of the evidence-based practice framework

acquire, appraise, apply and *assess*. Further development in the area noted that it was not enough to just assess the final research outcome, it was also important to disseminate the results for the betterment of the wider clinical community. Additionally, Melnyk and colleagues believed that no outcomes could be achieved, if there was not an initial research interest, which is sometimes referred to as Step Zero—the spirit of inquiry.[3] It is stressed that unless we encourage paramedics and paramedicine researchers to question current practice with ongoing research, our clinicians will not have the best evidence to play a vital role in the evidence-based medicine triad.

Example

A strong example to demonstrate the framework of evidence-based practice is the PARAMEDIC2 trial: investigating the effects of adrenaline on survival from out-of-hospital cardiac arrest (OHCA).

Starting with the 'spirit of inquiry', although the use of adrenaline in the treatment of OHCA is common, there was no definitive research to determine if adrenaline was actually helpful or harmful in OHCA. It was believed that although the use of adrenaline may be helpful in achieving a return of spontaneous circulation (ROSC), if may actually be detrimental to patient survival to the point of hospital discharge. This led to international interest in more definitive research in this area, which was supported by the International Liaison Committee on Resuscitation (ILCOR).

Together the research team determined the aim of their research, which would allow them to 'ask' the research question relevant to their concerns. According to the trial protocol, the primary objective of the trial was to determine the clinical effectiveness of adrenaline in the treatment of OHCA.[4] Once they had established their objective the team 'acquired' the current evidence to help confirm the need for the research. A part of the process also included 'appraise(ing)' the current evidence which did lead to the belief that there was not sufficient evidence to lead to clinical practice change recommendations in regards to the use of adrenaline in OHCA. The research team then 'apply(ied)' their research objective through the completion of the approved PARAMEDIC2 trial. The trial started in December 2014, after ethical approval was obtained and the trial was registered with the Clinical Trials Registry. Data collection continued for 3 years, at which time the researchers 'assess(ed)' their own results. In short, they found that although those who were given adrenaline compared to a placebo were slightly more likely to survive to 30 days after they had their OHCA (0.8% difference), those who were given the adrenaline were nearly twice as likely to have severe brain damage compared to those who had the placebo.[5]

After completing the 5 As, the research team 'disseminate(d)' their results to the research community, paramedics and the general wider community. This included peer-reviewed publications[5] and leaflets made available in multiple languages and audiences. Through this dissemination they have made it possible for ILCOR and ambulance services internationally to decide if they should change their guidelines, therefore leading to a shift in the research component in the evidence-based medicine triad.

STRENGTHS AND WEAKNESSES OF EVIDENCE-BASED PRACTICE

There are strengths and weakness to any approach to clinical care. For paramedics, although their clinical practice guidelines can be taken as the most relevant research, evidence-based practice helps them to take a holistic approach to patient care, acknowledging the wants of their patient and the clinician's own treatment recommendations based on their experience. However, there are also challenges in the paramedicine setting as research is still in its infancy. The available evidence may not be of the strongest quality or may not be specific to the out-of-hospital setting. This means that the paramedics may need to rely on their own experience and the patient's preferences to a greater extent, not fully working with the evidence-based practice triad balance. Regardless, accreditation boards view evidence-based practice as an important aspect of paramedic practice and have included it as one of five domains of professional capability for registered paramedics.[6]

CONCLUSION

Evidence-based practice encourages the clinician to equally rely on the best evidence, the patients wants and the clinician's own expertise when deciding on the best treatment plan for a patient. To do this successfully, research engaging with the evidence-based practice framework is required to help advise the development of clinical practice guidelines. Ongoing research in paramedicine will continue to diversify the relevant evidence, making it easier for paramedics to incorporate evidence-based practice into their clinical care.

REVIEW QUESTIONS

1. Are there examples in your own clinical practice that would have seen you implement evidence-based practice?
2. Are there areas in your service where you feel that the latest evidence may not align with your clinical practice guidelines? If so (or if there is no evidence), what do you think you can do as a paramedic to promote change?

SUGGESTED FURTHER READING

PARAMEDIC Trial Team. PARAMEDIC2: Should adrenaline be used when someone's heart stops? Coventry, UK: Warwick Clinical Trials Unit, Warwick Medical School, University of Warwick; 2018. Online. Available: https://warwick.ac.uk/fac/sci/med/research/ctu/trials/critical/paramedic2/.

REFERENCES

1. Sackett DL, Rosenberg WM, Gray JM, Haynes RB, Richardson WS. Evidence-based medicine: what it is and what it isn't. British Medical Journal Publishing Group; 1996.
2. National Health and Medical Research Council. Australian clinical practice guidelines. 2017. Online. Available: https://www.clinicalguidelines.gov.au/portal.
3. Melnyk BM, Fineout-Overholt E, Stillwell SB, Williamson KM. Evidence-based practice: step by step: the seven steps of evidence-based practice. American Journal of Nursing. 2010;110(1):51–3.
4. Perkins GD, Quinn T, Deakin CD, Nolan JP, Lall R, Slowther A-M, et al. Pre-hospital assessment of the role of adrenaline: measuring the effectiveness of drug administration in cardiac arrest (PARAMEDIC-2): trial protocol. Resuscitation. 2016;108:75–81.
5. Perkins GD, Ji C, Deakin CD, Quinn T, Nolan JP, Scomparin C, et al. A randomized trial of epinephrine in out-of-hospital cardiac arrest. New England Journal of Medicine. 2018;379(8):711–21.
6. Paramedicine Board Ahpra. Professional capabilities for registered paramedics. 2021. Online. Available: https://www.paramedicineboard.gov.au/professional-standards/professional-capabilities-for-registered-paramedics.aspx.

4

How to Use this Book

Kelly-Ann Bowles, Alexander Olaussen, Brett Williams and Bill Lord

LEARNING OUTCOMES

1. Develop a plan to use the contents of this book to provide a foundation for your understanding of research methods
2. Understand the gaps in your research knowledge to determine how to address them
3. Support your journey as a novice researcher

INTRODUCTION

The earlier chapters in this book have provided some insight into why paramedics must be involved in research. As has been discussed, the role of the paramedic has substantially changed over the last 20 years, and research has shown that in clinical areas where out-of-hospital interventions can occur, paramedics can have a significantly positive effect on patient outcomes. Where once expert opinion guided much of paramedicine, rigorously designed research has enabled the development of contemporary evidence-based practice guidelines. Further to this, much work has been completed to support the professionalisation of the paramedic profession, with strong agreement that structured education, with a large emphasis on tertiary education, has been paramount in the ongoing development of the profession. A knowledge of research methods that underpin the generation of discipline-specific data is a fundamental professional attribute.[1] Finally, by including paramedics in research, the complexities around conducting projects in the prehospital space can be identified and addressed, and the overall relevance of the research can be ensured. The aim of this book is therefore to provide foundational research skills to paramedics and those conducting or contemplating research in the paramedicine area.

Expanding on the learning objectives for this chapter, the aims of this book are to:

1. expose paramedics and paramedicine researchers to the broad range of research designs and approaches that they could use in their research

2. provide foundation-level information on selected research designs and approaches to help paramedics and paramedicine researchers decide which may be the best approach for them

3. present other information relevant to the research journey to support paramedics and paramedicine researchers to take their research idea from the initial question to the final dissemination/implementation.

As a number of research books suggest, the best way to use this book may involve reading sections more than once. The editors of the book have spent much time establishing a flow that is logical in the process of research design and completion. However, the novice researcher may not yet know the best approach for their project and therefore may need to review different sections to effectively 'find the best fit' for their work. This may mean reading the book initially in its entirety before you can focus your research question and then review the relevant sections. Going straight to the sections that you feel may be most relevant may do a disservice to your overall project if you have not considered other possible approaches. The selection of appropriate qualitative design is a good example.

However, this book is not designed to provide you with all the information you will require on a particular research design or approach. The book aims to provide a broad yet limited explanation of the research designs and approaches, along with further guidance on how to find additional in-depth information for a specific research project. It would be optimistic and perhaps unreasonable for any researcher to feel that they can obtain all of their education from one book, and it is only from using multiple resources (be that textbooks, publications, online learning and/or structured teaching as well as the advice of research experts), that we are truly able to cement our knowledge to ensure research rigour. Some suggestions have therefore been provided in the suggested further reading section in each chapter.

Finally, it is important to understand that research is a journey that is filled with constant learning. Many of you may be experts in your clinical space and have now taken yourself out of your comfort zone to learn about research. This can be daunting and at times you may feel very lost. This is normal. Do not feel that reading a chapter once will be enough to make everything perfectly clear to you. Starting research training is like taking yourself back to the first day you learned your clinical skills. You have learned the skills in some form of education, you practised them, learned from your mistakes and over time have developed a skill set that is now second nature to you. The same is possible with research.

CONCLUSION

Embarking on a research journey can be quite overwhelming as there is so much to consider and new processes to learn. Use this book to provide you with foundation information in your research education so that you can contribute to the expanding world of paramedicine research. Also remember to seek advice from experts who may be prepared to act as a research mentor.

REVIEW QUESTIONS

1. Consider your current knowledge about research designs. Have you thought about whether a different approach or design may give you a stronger answer to your question?
2. Do you have peers who have been involved in research? Can they provide insight into the best starting approach for them?
3. Do you have access to a 'research community'? Is there a university or learning institution that is completing research in your areas of interest that you could get involved in? Does your employer have a 'research team' that you could speak to?
4. Are there established researchers in a space you are interested in? It is worth reaching out as you would be surprised by the response you get.

REFERENCES

1. Reed B, Cowin L, O'Meara P, Wilson I. Professionalism and professionalisation in the discipline of paramedicine. Australasian Journal of Paramedicine. 2019;16:160. Online. Available: https://ajp.paramedics.org/index.php/ajp/article/view/715.

5

How to Determine What Topic to Research

Niamh M Cummins

LEARNING OUTCOMES

1. Define a research topic
2. Recognise the importance of choosing the right research topic
3. Identify the factors influencing the selection of a research topic

DEFINITION

A research topic is the subject or issue that a researcher is interested in exploring in their research project.

INTRODUCTION

Although it occurs early in the research process, determining what topic to research is one of the most challenging steps to overcome when undertaking a research project. Using a basic decision tree, like the example in Figure 5.1, can help get you started.

The diverse settings in which paramedics work offer a great opportunity for researchers to define their own research space, acknowledging that the out-of-hospital environment raises unique challenges not always seen in other health settings.[1] However, these issues are not unsurmountable, and because paramedicine is a young discipline there remain many gaps in the research evidence.[2] This means it is fertile ground for paramedicine researchers with a wide array of potential topics to be explored.[3] When selecting a research topic, it's best to start with a broad area and then narrow down your topic. This will later be refined to a research question which is specific and

defined, as discussed in the next chapter. At the conception stage of the research process, it is important to consider the significance of the work you aim to complete. Not all research projects need to make a large change to clinical practice, but all research needs to add to the current evidence. For example, this could be the application of an accepted treatment process in a new setting or the description of a clinical response that colleagues have been noticing more in the work. Either way, to ensure that our research can add to future change, we need to understand the current research in our space, carefully plan our project and ensure that correct processes are followed so that our findings can be useful for as many people as possible.

EXAMPLE

Although some paramedics find the idea of research daunting, the logical process of research development is not that different from the structure of a clinical primary and secondary survey. In the following example, these processes are aligned to demonstrate that paramedics are very well-equipped to complete research projects by implementing their structured approach to clinical assessment to that of the process of research. In the same way that paramedics

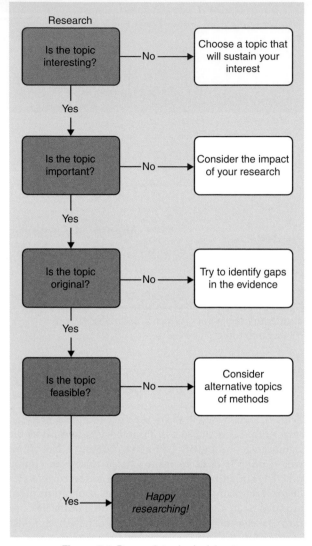

Figure 5.1 Research topic decision tree

assess the patient and scene when deciding on their treatment approach, in the following example the reader is challenged to think about their research environment when deciding which research topic to complete.

Primary Survey

A—Assessment

First, it's worth assessing yourself; think about your strengths and try to align your choice of research topic with those. What issues are you most passionate about? Choose a topic that you really enjoy and for your first project choose something that's achievable in a short timeframe

(e.g. 6 months). Consider also if there is a topic that's an area of interest in your service, local hospital or university.

B—Brainstorm

Where can you find inspiration for your research topic? This could come from your patients, colleagues, service organisation, clinical practice guidelines, the literature and so on. Are there current 'hot topics'? Talking to another professional in the field who has previously conducted research might also help to develop an idea and clarify your thinking. Create a 'mind map' of your ideas and always check that your question has its own unique aspect to add to the current evidence.

C—Collaborate

Similar to clinical care in the out-of-hospital setting, research is often improved when we work as a part of a team. Consider this when choosing your research topic. Have you identified a supervisor or mentor? Do you have colleagues who have conducted research before? Where can you find support: from your service, in-hospital colleagues, academic institution or professional body? Surround yourself with like-minded researchers! Ideally aim to engage a research team with each member having unique skills and at least one experienced member to guide the projects if challenges arise.

Secondary Survey

D—Data

Consider what data you will need to address your research topic? Do you want to answer a question with numbers (quantitative data) or do you want to understand the reasons why something may or may not have happened (qualitative data)? What methods will you use to collect your data? Are there validated tools available? If you're collecting patient data, is it easily accessible (e.g. electronic patient care reports [ePCR] versus paper records)?

E—Ethics

Ethics may impact your choice of research topic—will you require ethical approval to conduct your project? If so, where does this approval need to be obtained from? Does your service have a research committee and do you need this approval as well as ethics approval? Is institutional approval required from your local university or hospital? How long does this process take? Make sure you seek expert advice on ethics applications and take any support that is offered from human research ethics committees.

F—Funding and feasibility

Funding might not be necessary for your project—it is possible to conduct excellent research and remain 'cost-neutral' (e.g. conducting a review or an online survey)—but it is a consideration when choosing your research topic as you may have more options if you can obtain funding. Potential sources of funding include service organisations, state bodies, universities, industry and charitable foundations. For some areas, funding will be required or the completion of the project will not be feasible.

CONCLUSION

Choosing a research topic is an iterative process, and in order to select a suitable research topic, a large amount of preparation work needs to be completed first. Don't be disheartened if it takes a few attempts to find the right topic for you. This investment of time early on will reward you later in the process and could save you a lot of frustration and time in the long term. It's also completely normal to feel lost at the beginning of a research project. Research is a skill just like any other and practice makes perfect. Finally, choose a research topic that you are passionate about, and soon you'll be on your way to formulating your research question.

REVIEW QUESTIONS

1. Think about your strengths as a paramedic. How could these translate to research?

2. Consider the first idea that comes to mind as a research topic. Now think about the barriers and facilitators to you doing research on that topic and list these in order of importance.

SUGGESTED FURTHER READING

Wang GT, Park K. Student research and report writing: from topic selection to the complete paper. Wiley Blackwell; 2016.

REFERENCES

1. Maurin Söderholm H, Andersson H, Andersson Hagiwara M, Backlund P, Bergman J, Lundberg L, et al. Research challenges in prehospital care: the need for a simulation-based prehospital research laboratory. Advances in Simulation. 2019;4:3.
2. Jensen JL, Bigham BL, Blanchard IE, Dainty KN, Socha D, Carter A, et al. The Canadian National EMS Research Agenda: a mixed methods consensus study. Canadian Journal of Emergency Medicine. 2013;15(2):73–82.
3. Snooks H, Evans A, Wells B, Pcconi J, Thomas M, Woollard M, et al. What are the highest priorities for research in emergency prehospital care? Emergency Medicine Journal. 2009;26(8):549–50.

6

Asking the Answerable Question

Navindhra Naidoo

LEARNING OUTCOME

1. Identify frameworks that can assist in the formulation of answerable research questions for clinical or health policy

INTRODUCTION

Healthcare systems are faced with the challenge of improving the quality of care and decreasing the risk of adverse events. Evidence from clinical research is necessary but not sufficient for delivering optimal care. Knowledge translation (KT) is the scientific study of methods for closing the knowledge-to-practice gap, and of the barriers and facilitators inherent in this process.[1] Evidence-based practice (EBP) is predicated on a knowledge need that is articulated in a research question.[2] When undertaking any research, answerable questions are important to: 1. ensure you have the correct terminology so that you are confident that you have collated the previous research in the area; 2. help you establish your outcome measures and; 3. help others find your work once it is published.

FORMULATING THE CLINICAL QUESTION

The first step in the EBP process is to translate this need into a searchable and answerable question. This will help to focus on the key issues, identify what evidence is needed to answer the question and perform an efficient search for evidence.[3] Therefore, structuring and refining the question is crucial. There are a range of ways that researchers establish their question, guided by the research approach. Search mnemonics are helpful frameworks and memory aids to deconstruct questions into meaningful parts.

PICO (see Table 6.1), can provide a useful structure to guide the development of questions.[4] Think about your knowledge gap that you wish to address and identify the PICO components. You should then spend time reflecting on your components and confirm the relevance of your question. Questions can be constructed as: 'In P (population), how does an I (intervention), compared to a C (comparator), affect O (outcomes)?' For context: Among domestic violence survivors, how does universal screening by paramedics, compared to selective screening and clinical case finding, affect domestic violence detection and referral?

When one wishes to investigate the outcome measure at a specific time or duration, then PICOT, where T refers to time, may be prudent.[5] For example, certain outcome measures may be decidedly different pre/post COVID-19 (T) or after a scope of practice change. Therefore, PICOT can be replaced with PICOC (where C represents context) when the context for intervention delivery is relevant.[6] A variation to PICOT is PICOTT, where TT refers to the type of question and the best type of study design to answer that question.[7] The criticism (and value) of this framework is that it can be too restrictive and therefore miss relevant evidence. For each concept, identify related keywords and synonyms. To translate the PICO concept into an effective database search, the database features (such as subject headings and truncation) should be optimised.

PIPOH was specifically developed for building and adapting guidelines.[8] The second P refers to professionals to whom the guideline will be targeted, and H stands for healthcare setting and context in which the adapted

TABLE 6.1 The PICO Framework with the Components That Contribute to the Development of a Research Question

Acronym	Component	Definition	Example
P	Population	The population, patient or problem being addressed	Domestic violence survivors
I	Intervention	What main intervention or issue are you considering?	Universal screening
C	Comparison	What will the intervention or issue be compared to? (Not all questions will include a comparison.)	Selective screening and clinical case finding
O	Outcome	What outcome does the intervention or issue seek to accomplish, measure, improve or affect?	Domestic violence detection and referral

guideline will be used. An example of this in the paramedicine setting would be: 'What is appropriate mentorship training to improve the quality of emergency clinicians working as clinical mentors in an ambulance service?' (P – population: clinical mentors; I – intervention: mentorship training; P – professionals: emergency clinicians; O – outcome: quality improvement; H – setting: ambulance service).

HEALTH POLICY AND MANAGEMENT QUESTIONS

PICO and its variations were all developed to answer clinical questions. Emergency services are complex social organisations that need to be sustainable and accountable. ECLIPSE (see Table 6.2) is an alternate approach to developing questions to address the health policy and management area.[9] For example, assume there have been healthcare user complaints about the new ambulance service superstation response times. What alternatives might improve customer satisfaction?

FORMULATING QUALITATIVE QUESTIONS

Qualitative research takes on a different approach to quantitative research as the former generalises its findings towards a theory/explanation while the latter intends generalisation of findings towards a population. Qualitative questions may include: Sample, Phenomenon of Interest, Design, Evaluation and Research Type (SPIDER).[10] However, DiCenso, Guyatt and Ciliska (2005) suggested that questions which can best be answered with qualitative information require just two components (PS; see Table 6.3) that focus on the meaning of an experience or problem.[11] For example: 'In a public health service, should all emergency communication centre staff who have telephone contact with healthcare users attend a customer awareness course?'

While PICO is likely the most used acronym, it deliberately limits scope. Combining comparable and related terms would provide the following conceptual framework (see Table 6.4) for a wider range of applications.[12] The caveat is that not all aspects may be relevant to your question.

TABLE 6.2 The ECLIPSE Framework for Health Policy or Management Research Questions

Acronym	Component	Definition	Example
E	Expectation	Why does the user want the information?	Improve customer satisfaction
C	Client group	For whom is the service intended?	Healthcare users who request an ambulance
L	Location	Where is the service physically sited?	New superstation in location X
I	Impact	What is the service change being evaluated? What would represent success? How is this measured? This component is similar to outcomes of the PICO framework.	Improve the new superstation service response times (or expectation thereof)
P	Professionals	Who provides or improves the service?	Ambulance service staff
SE	Service	What type of service is under consideration?	Ambulance service

TABLE 6.3 **The PS Framework for Qualitative Research Questions**

Acronym	Component	Definition	Example
P	Population	The characteristics of individuals, families, groups or communities	Emergency communication centre staff with user contact
S	Situation	An understanding of the condition, experiences, circumstances or situation	Customer awareness course

TABLE 6.4 **Components that May Contribute to The Development of an Answerable Question**

Acronym	Component
P	Population or problem
I	Intervention or exposure
C	Comparison
O	Outcome
C	Context or environment or setting
P	Professionals
R	Research: incorporating type of question and type of study design Results
S	Stakeholder or perspective or potential users
T	Timeframe or duration

In applying the frameworks in this chapter, researchers will be asking a range of questions inherent in the frameworks to develop answerable questions. Should any framework not suit the question, then defaulting to an epidemiological approach may offer pragmatic relief by considering: What? Who? Why? When? Where? and How? Ensure your question has relevance and that the work you wish to embark on is ethical and feasible (consider time and budgetary limitations too). You (and the scientific community) should find your research interesting and novel. Lastly, the question must be epigrammatic (i.e. short, fully informative and succinct).[13]

CONCLUSION

These frameworks are useful tools to guide the search strategy formation. The different elements—timeframe, duration, context, (healthcare) setting, environment, type of question, type of study design, professionals, exposure,

esults, stakeholders and situation—are used interchangeably. Researchers are encouraged 'to refine strategies to suit each particular situation rather than trying to fit a search situation to a framework'.[12]

REVIEW QUESTIONS

Think about a research question that is of interest to you. Break that question down into the question's components.
1. Who is the population of interest?
2. Is there an intervention or exposure?
3. Is there something that we are comparing the intervention or exposure to?
4. Are there set outcomes we are interested in?
5. Is this research time sensitive (e.g. during COVID-19)?
6. Are there only certain types of research designs that I am interested in?

SUGGESTED FURTHER READING

Cooke A, Smith D, Booth A. Beyond PICO: the SPIDER tool for qualitative evidence synthesis. Qualitative Health Research. 2012;22(10):1435–43.

Langlois EV, Daniels K, Akl EA, editors. Evidence Synthesis for health policy and systems: a methods guide. Geneva: World Health Organization; 2018.

National Health and Medical Research Council. Guidelines for Guidelines: adopt, adapt or start from scratch. NHMRC; 2018. Online. Available: https://www.nhmrc.gov.au/guidelinesforguidelines/plan/adopt-adapt-or-start-scratch.

Straus SE, Richardson WS, Glasziou P, Haynes RB. Evidence-based medicine: how to practice and teach EBM. London: Elsevier; 2008.

REFERENCES

1. Strauss S, Tetroe J, Graham ID, editors. Knowledge translation in health care. 2nd ed. New Jersey: Wiley-Blackwell; 2013.
2. Del Mar C, Hoffmann T, Glasziou P. Information needs, asking questions, and some basics of research studies. In: Hoffmann T, Del Mar C, Bennett S, editors. Evidence-based practice across

the health professions. Chatswood, NSW: Elsevier Australia; 2013, pp. 16–37.

3. LaTrobe University Library. Evidence-based practice in health. LaTrobe University. 2022. Online. Available: https://latrobe. libguides.com/ebp/Ask

4. Richardson WS, Wilson MC, Nishikawa J, Hayward RSA. The well-built clinical question: A key to evidence-based decisions. ACP Journal Club. 1995;123:A12–13.

5. Fineout-Overholt E, Johnson L. Teaching EBP: asking searchable, answerable clinical questions. Worldviews on Evidence-Based Nursing. 2005;2(3):157–60. http://doi.org/10.1111/j.1741-6787.2005.00032.x.

6. Petticrew M, Roberts H. Systematic reviews in the social sciences: a practical guide. Malden, MA: Blackwell Publishing; 2005

7. Schardt C, Adams MB, Owens T, Keitz S, Fontelo P. Utilization of the PICO framework to improve searching PubMed for clinical questions. BMC Medical Informatics and Decision Making. 2007;7:16. http://doi.org/10.1186/1472-6947-7-16.

8. Fervers B, Burgers JS, Voellinger R, Brouwers M, Browman GP, Graham ID, et al. ADAPTE Collaboration. Guideline adaptation: an approach to enhance efficiency in guideline development and improve utilisation. BMJ Quality & Safety. 2011 Mar;20(3):228–36. Epub 2011 Jan 5. PMID: 21209134. https://pubmed.ncbi.nlm.nih.gov/21209134/

9. Wildridge V, Bell L. How CLIP became ECLIPSE: a mnemonic to assist in searching for health policy/management information. Health Information and Libraries Journal. 2002;19(2): 113–15. http://doi.org/10.1046/j.1471-1842.2002.00378.x.

10. Cooke A, Smith D, Booth A. Beyond PICO: the SPIDER tool for qualitative evidence synthesis. Qualitative Health Research. 2012;22(10):1435–43.

11. DiCenso A, Guyatt G, Ciliska D. Evidence-based nursing: a guide to clinical practice. St Louis, MO: Elsevier Mosby; 2005.

12. Davies K. Formulating the evidence based practice question: a review of the frameworks. Evidence Based Library and Information Practice. 2011;6(2).

13. Aldous C, Rheeder P, Esterhuizen T. Writing your first clinical research protocol. Cape Town: Juta; 2011.

7

What to do Before You Start

Brendan Shannon and Alexander Olaussen

LEARNING OUTCOMES

1. Describe common pitfalls encountered in the early stages of research design
2. Identify the factors that lead to successful research project completion
3. Describe the key stakeholders required to be involved in the research and why their approval and engagement is often needed

INTRODUCTION

The best research questions start with a curious mind. Research questions from paramedics and paramedic students usually come about due to one or more of the following circumstances that are all underpinned by curiosity.

- A paramedic/student is confronted with a clinical conundrum that has forced them to wonder if they are currently doing things in the best way possible. You may be aware of interventions or processes being used in different settings that would help in the area you are currently working/training in, and your curiosity causes you to investigate further.
- A paramedic may be frustrated with something in their practice. It may be a systems process or intervention (or lack of intervention) that they feel is necessary to adjust in order to improve their working conditions or patient care.
- There may be a grant opportunity to look at something specific or a paramedic/student may be inspired to research an area that someone else would like investigated. These grants can come from academic supervisors or external stakeholders such as ambulance services, health services or other professional bodies.

Once you have what you feel is a great idea for research further, you may feel it's the most important thing since the discovery of fire. Your passion at this stage is important but to do things properly and reduce episodes of disappointment, we need to take a step back and think about some of the essential steps we need to undertake in order to do well. We suggest seven key steps to consider when starting out on your research journey, which complements Chapter 5 and the ABCDEF approach.

THE STEPS TO GETTING STARTED SUCCESSFULLY

Step 1: Ask Around / Get Feedback

The first step is to ask around. Seek out experts in the field that are accessible to you. This may mean reaching out to universities or researchers within your area of work who may have relevant expertise. If your initial contact person is not the right person to speak to, fear not—they will more than likely point you to someone who can help. You should run your ideas past these people and get feedback on your idea. Be prepared for feedback and embrace criticism. The following are key questions to ask.

- Is this a good idea or is there need for research from their perspective?
- Has this already been investigated or is it currently being investigated?
- Is it feasible to investigate this area and is there interest from key stakeholders?

Step 2: See What's Out There

If the early discussions show that your research idea is feasible, it's now time to do an environmental scan to see what already exists in both published and grey literature.[1] This is separate initially to a formal review; this will come later. The point of this environmental scan is to become familiar with the key ideas, concepts and trajectory of what's being done in the area of your research topic. At this stage it's important to keep a record of your ideas. This may include key phrases, key documents and literature that are informing your opinion. These early stages and recording your thoughts will help immensely when it comes to formulating and then refining your research question. Chapters 11 to 15 go through formal processes in searching the literature.

Step 3: Ask the Question

Now it's time to sit down and really flesh out your answerable research question. This will likely develop with input from others but it is important to start somewhere. Chapter 6 covers how to build an answerable question using the PICO format.[2] The first draft of your question is what you will now take to share with key stakeholders to get their involvement and critique.

Step 4: Get Stakeholders Involved

One of the first stakeholders you should get involved is a research mentor. A good mentor who brings out your strengths and points you in the right direction when needed and brings you up when you fall down is worth their weight in gold. Research is likely a completely new discipline for you and in the same way you need educators to guide you in your early clinical years, you need good research mentors and teachers. The next key stakeholder needed will likely be a health service or ambulance service. It's crucial you have in-principle support from all stakeholders for your research otherwise even the greatest research ideas and proposals can be stalled or at worst never move beyond the planning stage.

Step 5: Figure out How to Do It. What Design are You Going to Use?

Once you have a key mentor or two and some in-principle support or interest from those key stakeholders needed to undertake your research, it's time to start planning.[3] Proper preparation is key, and you need to be very critical of your approach to research at this stage in order to have success long term. Consider the following in choosing what design or process you will undertake.

- Are my questions associated with answering the what or the why? This will dictate what broad methodology you should follow in designing your research.
- Consideration of restraints:
  - Do you have deadlines that must be met? A randomised control trial may be a great method to answer the question, but can you wait years for your results?
  - Do you have or could you likely secure funding to support the costs associated with your research?

- Do you have expertise within your research team to undertake the research question and process? You should have people with clinical expertise/experience as their insight is important. You should also have those with research experience in your chosen methodology on your research team.
- Lastly and most importantly, is the research method ethical and have you considered all ethical implications of undertaking your research?

Step 6: Discuss Expectations, Both of Your Supervisor and Yourself

By this stage it's likely you have a solid plan for moving forward with your research topic, including an answerable question, buy-in from key stakeholders and a mentor(s) to guide you through the process. Now it's time to set out what is expected of you and also what you expect from your mentor(s).[4] This can be a formalised document or something else but at a minimum it's important to communicate these expectations from both parties clearly from the start to ensure everyone is on the same page. The importance of these discussions cannot be understated so please ensure you have them.

Step 7: Begin—and Don't Forget to Write

Now it's time to get started! Usually this will begin with some form of literature review (see Part 3 for more detail) and then writing a formal proposal. We would suggest writing early and often as no first draft is ever perfect. Remember that a poor draft can be edited, whereas a blank page cannot. Starting to write is key.[5]

CONCLUSION

The first step in starting research is often the most overwhelming. Hopefully by following the steps in this chapter you are set up for as much success as possible. The subsequent chapters in this book will guide you through the process of research, which when you peel it all back, is not as hard as it may seem at the beginning. Good luck!

REVIEW QUESTIONS

1. What is the difference between a concept, a theory and a theoretical framework?
2. Consider how and through which avenues you could reach out to paramedics in your network to discuss your research idea.
3. With a research question in mind, consider all the possible methodologies you could use to answer your question (e.g. literature review, different types of qualitative, quantitative and mixed methods techniques).

REFERENCES

1. Charlton P, Doucet S, Azar R, Nagel DA, Boulos L, Luke A, et al. The use of the environmental scan in health services delivery research: a scoping review protocol. BMJ Open. 2019;9(9):e029805.
2. Hastings C, Fisher CA. Searching for proof: creating and using an actionable PICO question. Nursing Management. 2014;45(8):9–12.
3. Ratan SK, Anand T, Ratan J. Formulation of research question—stepwise approach. Journal of Indian Association of Pediatric Surgeons. 2019;24(1):15.
4. Woolhouse M. Supervising dissertation projects: expectations of supervisors and students. Innovations in Education and Teaching International. 2002;39(2):137–44.
5. Kearns H, Gardiner M, Marshall K. Innovation in PhD completion: the hardy shall succeed (and be happy!). Higher Education Research & Development. 2008;27(1):77–89.

8

Theoretical and Conceptual Frameworks for Paramedicine Research

Alan M Batt and Madison Brydges

LEARNING OUTCOMES

1. Define and differentiate between a theory, theoretical framework and conceptual framework
2. Outline the benefits of using theoretical and/or conceptual frameworks in the design and conduct of a research study
3. Describe the practical first steps to engaging with theories, theoretical frameworks and conceptual frameworks in your research study

INTRODUCTION

While 'theory', 'theoretical framework' and 'conceptual framework' may be *familiar* terms, many readers may not *understand* them well. The landscape of theories and conceptual frameworks is complex, ever-expanding and challenging to navigate. Academic disciplines create and use theories and conceptual frameworks in different ways. The terms are often poorly articulated or discussed ambiguously, and consequently researchers may be hesitant to engage with them. The terms are also challenging to write about when constrained by the word limits of some scientific journals.

In this chapter, we will begin by exploring each term, providing some practical examples and finally highlighting considerations for using them in research.

DEFINING THE TERMS

Concepts are abstract ideas that together make up the 'building blocks' of theories.[1] An example is the concept of 'agency', which is the capacity of individuals to act independently and to make their own free choices. Theories describe how concepts are related in a way that explains the situation or phenomenon.[1] Theories have different aims, such as being descriptive, emancipatory, disruptive or predictive. Theories can explain large societal patterns or individual-level interactions.

Theoretical frameworks are logically developed and connected sets of concepts and theories that researchers create to scaffold a study.[1]

Conceptual frameworks represent the way we think about a problem or a study.[2] They justify why the research should be done by describing the state of known knowledge, identifying knowledge gaps and inform the methodology needed to study the problem.[1]

WHY CONSIDER THE USE OF THEORIES, THEORETICAL FRAMEWORKS AND CONCEPTUAL FRAMEWORKS?

Paramedicine research would be enhanced by further engaging with theories, theoretical frameworks and/or conceptual frameworks. Doing so enhances a researcher's ability to use their findings (related to a specific problem or phenomenon) to contribute to knowledge in a broader field of study. Theoretical and conceptual frameworks also have implications for methodology, such as the choice of an inductive (where you begin with observations that then allow you to develop or test a theory) or deductive (where you begin with a theory and test it with observations) approach.[1,3] Including theories and concepts in your research also helps readers to understand the methodological choices made during the research.[4]

EXAMPLE: THEORETICAL FRAMEWORK TO INFORM DEDUCTIVE STUDY

You are interested in whether paramedics have situational awareness and how this can be taught. You review the literature on situational awareness,[5] and identify several theories. While reviewing the different theories, you note that Endsley's theory of situational awareness appears to be an ideal framework.[6] Why? While all the theories explore situational awareness, Endsley's theory appears more comprehensive, separates the outcome from the process of having situational awareness and facilitates the measurement of decision-making and feedback (e.g. offers insights into areas for improvement in education). You begin the research by making three assumptions before using this theory: a paramedic would need to identify a situation accurately; the paramedic would need to interpret its meaning; and the paramedic would need to predict how the situation might unfold. You now use this theory as a framework and use the assumptions to inform your methodology and analysis plan.[7]

EXAMPLE: CONCEPTUAL FRAMEWORK TO STRUCTURE AN INDUCTIVE STUDY OF PARAMEDIC ROLE

You are interested in exploring how paramedics play a role in providing healthcare to those experiencing homelessness. Your research supervisor suggests you examine this topic from a constructivist approach, as it is an approach that embraces people's subjective lived experiences. From this starting point, you undertake a literature review to help further clarify your conceptual framework.

You review the literature on the role of paramedics in society, and this appears to be an understudied topic in paramedicine. You find a paper that conceptualises and describes paramedics' roles.[8] Considering the conceptual model outlined by Tavares and colleagues in this paper, you begin to wonder how and why paramedics may view themselves as 'health and social advocates', such as when providing patient care to those experiencing homelessness. You use this concept to narrow down your research question: what are paramedics' views on providing care to homeless populations? You design a study that will interview paramedics about their experiences providing care to those experiencing homelessness. Your analytical approach will be inductive, allowing the findings to be driven from the research participants' perspective.

PRACTICAL ADVICE

Using theories, concepts and theoretical frameworks is a challenge. We encourage all paramedicine researchers to start by asking for help from those with experience navigating this challenging research activity. Reading broadly, from within and outside of paramedicine, will help expose you to concepts and theories that may be useful.

It is helpful to draw on examples of research that clearly discusses *how* and *why* they have used theory. We have included some examples in Table 8.1. Focus on building connections between the literature, theory and concepts to develop your theoretical and conceptual framework. In your own work, clearly articulate which approach you took, why you made this choice and its implications.

CONCLUSION

Understanding the terms theory, theoretical frameworks and conceptual frameworks is challenging. Researchers approach and use these in different ways, making it important to clearly articulate the approach what was used in the research.

TABLE 8.1 **Examples of Research Studies Explicit in Their Use of Theory and Conceptual Frameworks**
Corman MK. Paramedics on and off the streets: emergency medical services in the age of technological governance. University of Toronto Press; 2017.
McCann L, Granter E, Hyde P, Hassard J. Still blue-collar after all these years? An ethnography of the professionalization of emergency ambulance work. Journal of Management Studies. 2013;50(5):750–76.
Rees N, Porter A, Rapport F, Hughes S, John A. Paramedics' perceptions of the care they provide to people who self-harm: a qualitative study using evolved grounded theory methodology. PLoS ONE. 2018;13(10):1–16. Online. Available: https://doi.org/10.1371/journal.pone.0205813.
Seim J. Bandage, sort, and hustle: ambulance crews on the front lines of urban suffering. University of California Press; 2020.

REVIEW QUESTIONS

1. What is the difference between a concept, a theory and a theoretical framework?
2. What are the benefits to your research of engaging with a theory or framework?
3. Can you identify challenges you may face in engaging with these suggestions?

REFERENCES

1. Varpio L, Paradis E, Uijtdehaage S, Young M. The distinctions between theory, theoretical framework and conceptual framework. Academic Medicine. 2020 Jul;95(7):989–94.
2. Bordage G. Conceptual frameworks to illuminate and magnify. Medical Education. 2009;43(4):312–9.
3. Timmermans S, Tavory I. Theory construction in qualitative research: from grounded theory to abductive analysis. Sociological Theory. 2012;30(3):167–86.
4. Maxwell JA. Conceptual framework: what do you think is going on? Qualitative research design: an interactive approach. 3rd ed. SAGE Publications; 2012, pp. 39–72.
5. Hunter J, Porter M, Williams B. What is known about situational awareness in paramedicine? A scoping review. Journal of Allied Health. 2019;48(1):e27–34.
6. Hunter J, Porter M, Williams B. Towards a theoretical framework for situational awareness in paramedicine. Safety Science. 2020; 122(January):104528.
7. Hunter J, Porter M, Phillips A, Evans-brave M, Williams B. Do paramedic students have situational awareness during high-fidelity simulation? A mixed-methods pilot study. International Emergency Nursing. 2021;56(February):100983.
8. Tavares W, Bowles R, Donelon B. Informing a Canadian paramedic profile: framing concepts, roles and crosscutting themes. BMC Health Services Research. 2016;16(1):1–16.

9

Overview of Research Designs and the Hierarchy of Evidence

Cameron M Gosling

LEARNING OUTCOMES

1. Understand levels of evidence and how the choice of design influences its strength

2. Identify and describe types of observational and experimental research designs

INTRODUCTION

The paramedicine researcher has many quantitative research design options to investigate the problem at hand. Often it is about a best-fit design to answer your research question, rather than the perfect design. The hierarchy of evidence provides an opportunity for novice researchers to understand the strength of designs selected and balance against the inherent biases within those designs before proceeding.

HIERARCHY OF EVIDENCE PYRAMID

The pyramid shown in Figure 9.1 is a graphical representation of the 'trade-off' between the quality of the evidence generated by each quantitative research design and the bias that would be found in each of those research designs. As the pyramid ascends towards a peak, the bias in research design declines; however, this evidence increases in quality as the designs become more robust. The greatest available evidence is for meta-analyses and systematic reviews of randomised controlled trials, increasing the confidence that significant results indicate causal relationships.

CASE STUDY/CASE SERIES

These studies are sometimes called a case report, and are often seen with new and emerging events, such as the early emergence of the COVID-19 virus. Case studies are detailed reports by one or more health professionals on the profile of a single patient and/or adverse event, particularly those that are rare in nature. Alternatively, a case series is a report on a series of patients with an outcome of interest. In these studies, there is generally no comparison group and they are deemed to be hypothesis generating. More detailed information, including relevant examples, can be found in Chapter 23.

ECOLOGICAL STUDY

An ecological, or correlation, study is where the units of analysis are populations or groups of people, rather than individuals. These designs are often used to compare disease frequencies between different populations during the same period of time, or between the same population at different time periods.

CROSS-SECTIONAL STUDY

Cross-sectional designs are similar to ecological, but we are now looking at individuals instead of populations. In a cross-sectional study, the units of analysis are individuals and are utilised to measure prevalence of disease and measures of exposure. Both disease and exposure can be assessed at the same point in time in a cross-sectional study. These study designs are good for establishing prevalence, which is the proportion of individuals with the outcome of

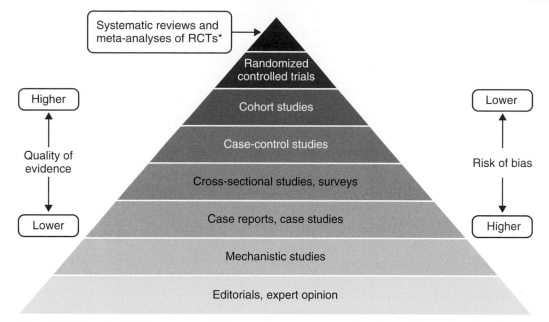

Figure 9.1 Hierarchy of evidence pyramid. *Meta-analyses and systematic reviews of observational studies and mechanistic studies are also possible. RCTs (randomised controlled trials). (Source: Yetley EA, MacFarlane AJ, Greene-Finestone LS, Garza C, Ard JD, Atkinson SA, et al. Options for basing Dietary Reference Intakes (DRIs) on chronic disease endpoints: report from a joint US-/Canadian-sponsored working group. The American Journal of Clinical Nutrition. 2017 Jan;105(1):249S–285S. Online. Available: https://doi.org/10.3945/ajcn.116.139097.)

interest at a particular point of time. Questionnaires taken at one time point are often cross-sectional studies. Further information on cross-sectional study designs is provided in Chapter 24.

CASE-CONTROL STUDY

A case-control study design is an effective method for the investigation of rare diseases or outcomes. These designs compare the occurrence of possible causes of an outcome in cases (someone who develops a condition) and controls (someone who does not develop the condition) where data of that outcome is collected at one point in time. The exposures experienced by the participants are collected at a previous point in time. In this respect, these designs are retrospective as the investigator is looking backward from the disease or outcome to identify possible causes. This design is often used in research looking at factors that may lead to cancer risk factors, where the researcher will compare factors in people who have developed cancer with people who have not developed cancer. Chapter 25 provides further insights into the use of case-control designs.

COHORT STUDY

A cohort study design can be observational and analytical. These designs 'allow nature to take its course' where the cohort with a common characteristic is followed. These study designs may also use a control, or comparison, group and data may be tracked prospectively or retrospectively. The incidence of an outcome is compared in participants selected on the basis of a shared characteristic between those exposed and those not exposed to a risk factor during the study time. Participants are then followed up to identify whether or not they have developed the outcome of interest. Cohort designs can provide good evidence of cause-and-effect relationships and are described in more detail in Chapter 26.

RANDOMISED CONTROLLED TRIAL (RCT)

The effects of an intervention are measured by comparing the outcomes in the group you have intervened with (experimental group) with that of the group you haven't intervened with (control group). RCTs are the 'gold standard' design for studying cause-and-effect relationships and are the cornerstone of evidence-based medicine. RCTs use tightly controlled study environments to limit external influences where participants are allocated to treatment/intervention or control/placebo groups using a random mechanism. Participants have an equal chance of being allocated to an intervention or control group. RCTs are covered in more detail in Chapter 27.

SYSTEMATIC REVIEWS AND META-ANALYSES

A systematic review is a methodology designed to identify, review, appraise and assimilate all available evidence on a research question. A systematic review may be narrative or analytical in nature, but is approached using a systematic method aimed at minimising bias. A meta-analysis generally uses the pooled results of RCTs to derive an overall conclusion for a defined question. The strength of these designs is the expansive search strategy, assessment of study quality and the more precise estimate of the effect of the intervention on the outcome of interest. Systematic reviews and meta-analyses are discussed in Chapter 15.

CONCLUSION

The type of design selected by a researcher is dependent on the structure of the research question. Once the question has been established, it is imperative a design is selected that maximises the quality of evidence collected while minimising any inherent biases. Other aspects should be considered when selecting the best design for your research, including ethical consideration. A useful tool to remember as a researcher is the hierarchy of evidence pyramid, which provides an easily referenced visual schema to aid in methodological selection.

REVIEW QUESTIONS

1. In your clinical work you have noticed that a small number of your patients are responding in an unusual way to medications in the month after an out-of-hospital cardiac arrest. What may be an initial way for you to share this finding with your colleagues?
2. A current clinical practice guideline feels dated and is possibly leading to further harm for patients. What may be a good way to produce evidence to inform a clinical practice guideline change?

SUGGESTED FURTHER READING

Cochrane Training. Evidence Essentials. Online. Available: https://training.cochrane.org/essentials.

Thinking About Ethics in Research

Paul Simpson and Susan Furness

LEARNING OUTCOMES

1. Summarise the four principles governing human research ethics

2. Describe the key ethics frameworks relevant to human research ethics

INTRODUCTION

Recent decades have seen a rapid expansion of paramedicine research as paramedics continue to establish a body of evidence to describe, support and evolve the discipline.[1] Irrespective of the type of research being conducted, consideration of ethical issues presents the same challenges faced by researchers in other healthcare disciplines. While research ethics frameworks and guidance exist, application of these to the dynamic emergency context of paramedicine can be difficult.[2] A paramedicine researcher can best prepare themselves for managing ethical considerations by developing a strong grounding in the broad foundational principles underpinning all human research in healthcare. In this chapter, we provide an orientation to research governance and ethics frameworks and an overview of general principles and values central to ethical research practice.

THE ORIGINS OF HUMAN RESEARCH ETHICS AND CONTEMPORARY FRAMEWORKS

Research ethics were brought into sharp focus in the aftermath of World War II when the Nuremberg trials were convened to investigate systematic abuse of marginalised persons through research experimentation, leading to the creation and adoption of the Nuremburg Code.[3] In 1964 the World Medical Assembly adopted the Declaration of Helsinki, which outlines ethical principles for human medical research. The most recent version of this policy is available on the World Medical Assembly website (see the Further reading section of this chapter), and remains the cornerstone on which contemporary human research guidelines are created.

Using these cornerstone statements, most countries developed their own frameworks adapted to specific needs. For example, in Australia, research is governed by the Australian Code for the Responsible Conduct of Research, collaboratively produced by the National Health and Medical Research Council (NHMRC), the Australian Research Council (ARC) and Universities Australia (UA).[4] That same collaboration also produced the National Statement on Ethical Conduct in Human Research to guide research stakeholders on ethical considerations.[5]

THE PRINCIPLES AND VALUES OF HUMAN RESEARCH ETHICS

The following describes four core research values (see Figure 10.1) that should guide the ethical design, review and conduct of human research.[5]

- Research merit and integrity
  - Research should have merit, in that its conduct is necessary and that the benefits arising from it to participants or society more broadly outweigh the risk arising from the research.
  - Research should be rigorous in design and methodology, informed by literature and be supervised by appropriately experienced people.

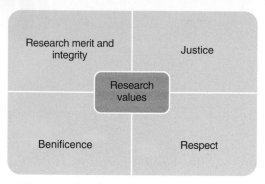

Figure 10.1 The principles and values underpinning research ethics[5]

- Justice
  - Fairness should exist in relation to inclusion and/or exclusion of participants; recruitment; access to benefits of research.
  - Research should be free of exploitation of particular participants, groups or cultures.
  - There should be fairness in reporting and dissemination of findings relating to participants or participant groups.
- Beneficence
  - The potential benefits arising from the research justify any potential harms.
  - Research should be designed to minimise the risk of harm or discomfort to participants.
  - Participants should be clearly aware of risk associated with their participation.
  - Research should include a mechanism to monitor participant welfare and intervene if required.
- Respect
  - Research must respect the privacy, confidentiality and cultural sensitivities of participants.
  - Research must respect and value the fundamental human right to self-determination, autonomy and capacity to make one's own decisions.
  - Respect the principle of choice regarding participation and protect those whose ability to choose may be compromised or may be lacking in capacity.

ETHICS APPROVAL PROCESSES

Ethical review of proposed research projects is the responsibility of human research ethics committees (HRECs). Most commonly, researchers will engage with a HREC within a university; however, many healthcare services also have a HREC or equivalent committee able to provide ethical approval for research being done under that service's auspices. Once ethical approval has been granted by a HREC, there may be a requirement for the researcher to then pursue a second layer of approval, known as 'site-specific approval', from a governance committee embedded within the health service in which the proposed research it to take place.

The process for seeking ethical review of a proposed project is fairly consistent across locations and organisations, although specific requirements may vary from site to site. HRECs have clearly defined ethical review pathways; the paramedicine researcher is encouraged to engage with the relevant research governance officer at the selected institution early in the research development phase to facilitate an efficient review process. Early decisions revolve around initial assessment of risk based on the proposed study protocol. Levels of risk can be categorised as follows.[5]

- Negligible risk: There is no foreseeable risk of harm or discomfort and any foreseeable risk is no more than inconvenience.
- Low risk: The maximum foreseeable risk is discomfort.
- Greater than low risk: The foreseeable risk is greater than discomfort.

There are instances in which ethical approval may not be required such as quality assurance or improvement, or clinical audit. The line between what constitutes 'research' as opposed to 'quality improvement', 'evaluation' or 'audit' can be difficult to discern, with the NHMRC suggesting these exist on a continuum of activity.[6] The latter usually sit on the low-to-negligible risk level, and so may be exempted from requiring HREC approval. That does not mean assessment of ethical considerations is not required; most institutions will have an internal governance committee below the level of a HREC that will conduct review of quality insurance, evaluation or audit projects to ensure adherence to broad ethical principles.[6]

While the ethics approval process can at times feel onerous, the process is fundamental to ensuring that research values are upheld, and participants are treated in a safe, ethical and responsible manner (see Box 10.1).

BOX 10.1   Key Point

Gaining ethical approval for research is a vital step on the path to commencing a project. The approval process must not be seen as an inconvenient administrative hurdle in the cycle of research, required only for future acceptance of the study in a journal. It should be viewed as a critical component of research design collaboratively reviewed and managed by the research team and a HREC/REC.

APPLIED EXAMPLE 1

Melanie is a paramedic and lead investigator on a research project involving paramedicine students. She is having difficulty reaching her target participant quota and is keen to enlist more participants. She approaches the student group to encourage involvement, stating: 'I know your coordinator and will inform them of your unprofessional and uncaring attitude if you don't agree to participate'.

Melanie uses coercion to improve participation, and the ethical principle of respect in regard to self-determination, autonomy and capacity has been breached. This example also demonstrates a lack of research integrity. Ethics applications should clearly outline how participants will be recruited, and these need to be adhered to at all stages of the research process. Consideration should also be given to the management of existing power dynamics between the researcher and participants.

APPLIED EXAMPLE 2

Rasheed is a paramedicine researcher conducting qualitative research exploring help-seeking behaviours of paramedics experiencing challenges to their mental health. During interviews Rasheed believes there to be a risk that participants could become distressed or anxious as they discuss sensitive content. Within the research protocol, Rasheed incorporates consideration of participant wellness by providing participants with links to pastoral support infrastructure. She makes this risk clear and evident in the participant information sheet so that paramedics can make an informed decision regarding participation.

Rasheed is adhering to core research values, specifically beneficence. Researchers must ensure participants are well informed as the potential harms associated with participation in a project, and the likelihood of those harms occurring. Further, it is the responsibility of the researcher to implement appropriate harm-mitigation measures designed to protect participants and support them if harm occurs.

APPLIED EXAMPLE 3

A randomised controlled trial (RCT) conducted in the United Kingdom sought to investigate the impact of adrenaline, compared to placebo, on survival from out-of-hospital cardiac arrest (OOHCA).[7] The patients to be enrolled in the study had experienced a cardiac arrest and would be unable to provide informed consent to participate. As the study commenced, an aggressive publicity campaign was rolled out in the regions in which the research would take place to inform the population from which participants might be drawn.[7] They introduced a prospective 'opt-out' system in which people could register their refusal to participate. The research team were granted a 'waiver of consent' by a HREC, allowing for a patient to be enrolled in a time-critical emergency resuscitation situation. As soon as practicable after the initial emergency had passed, the researchers approached patients or their legal representative and informed them of their participation and request consent to continue including them in the trial.[8]

The researchers went to extraordinary lengths to inform prospective patients about the study, even so far as implementing an opt-out system. Despite the waiver of consent, they still sought to gain consent in a pragmatic way from relatives or legal representatives later, without compromising the provision of care at the time of the incident. Thus, the researchers sought to adhere as best as the context allowed to the principles of research merit and integrity, justice and respect. It is worth noting that the approval of waived consent in this study triggered significant debate among ethicists, researchers, the public and the paramedics providing the initial care.[8, 9] The paramedics themselves reported feeling challenged in an ethical and moral sense, a phenomenon documented in earlier paramedicine research.[8,10] The case illustrates the complexity of the ethical considerations that surround the conduct of prospective clinical research on patients in the emergency care setting.[11]

CONCLUSION

By engaging in the careful analysis of ethical considerations during the design phase of a research project, a paramedicine researcher can be sure of conducting research that upholds the core values and principles of human research ethics. Critical discussion of ethical considerations should be guided by recognised research ethics statements relevant to the locality in which the research will conducted.

REVIEW QUESTIONS

1. A colleague approaches you about partnering in writing a literature review for publication in a peer-reviewed journal. She states it will be either a systematic review or a scoping review. Will you need to seek approval from a human research ethics committee (HREC) for the proposed project? Provide a justification for your position.

2. You are part of a research team that is planning to investigate the experiences of patients who have chest pain and receive care from paramedics. Your colleague proposes that patient consent be gained at the scene during treatment, prior to transport being initiated, arguing that this will increase the number of patients who agree

to participate without compromising patient care. Apply the four key principles of research ethics to this situation and analyse the appropriateness of the planned recruitment process.

3. You have designed an online survey to investigate the experiences of paramedics who have had to make decisions to terminate resuscitation in the out-of-hospital setting. The survey will ask participants to reflect on such cases discuss how these encounters made them feel during and after the incident. It will be completed anonymously by registered paramedics. You advise your co-researchers that the ethics approval will be simple given the project has a low to negligible risk. One of your colleagues disagrees, and asks you to reconsider your position. Analyse the project, identifying the potential harms of discomforts that may exist and revisit your risk assessment. Will it be viewed as low-to-negligible risk by a HREC? Justify your position.

SUGGESTED FURTHER READING

World Medical Association Declaration of Helsinki—Ethical Principles for Medical Research Involving Human Subjects. Online. Available: https://www.wma.net/policies-post/wma-declaration-of-helsinki-ethical-principles-for-medical-research-involving-human-subjects/.

REFERENCES

1. Simpson P. Quantifying and evaluating research in paramedicine—why our own field of research code matters. Australasian Journal of Paramedicine. 2020;17.

2. Armstrong S, Langlois A, Siriwardena N, Quinn T. Ethical considerations in prehospital ambulance based research: qualitative interview study of expert informants. BMC Medical Ethics. 2019;20(1):1–12.

3. Lahman MK, Geist MR, Rodriguez KL, Graglia P, DeRoche KK. Culturally responsive relational reflexive ethics in research: the three Rs. Quality & Quantity. 2011;45(6):139–414.

4. National Health and Medical Research Council, Australian Research Council and Universities Australia. Australian code for the responsible conduct of research. 2018. Canberra: Commonwealth of Australia.

5. National Health and Medical Research Council, Australian Research Council and Universities Australia. National statement on ethical conduct in human research. 2018. Canberra: Commonwealth of Australia.

6. National Health and Medical Research Council. Ethical considerations in quality assurance and evaluation activities. 2014. Online. Available: https://www.nhmrc.gov.au/about-us/resources/ethical-considerations-quality-assurance-and-evaluation-activities.

7. Perkins GD, Ji C, Deakin CD, Quinn T, et al. A randomized trial of epinephrine in out-of-hospital cardiac arrest. New England Journal of Medicine. 2018;379(8):711–21.

8. Charlton K, Franklin J, McNaughton R. Phenomenological study exploring ethics in prehospital research from the paramedic's perspective: experiences from the Paramedic-2 trial in a UK ambulance service. Emergency Medicine Journal. 2019;36(9):535–40.

9. McCartney M. Adrenaline in cardiac arrest: it's unethical for patients not to know. BMJ. 2014;349.

10. Hargreaves K, Goodacre S, Mortimer P. Paramedic perceptions of the feasibility and practicalities of prehospital clinical trials: a questionnaire survey. Emergency Medicine Journal. 2014;31(6):499–504.

11. Moscati R. Protection of human subjects in prehospital research. Prehospital Emergency Care. 2002;6(sup2):S18–23.

Preparing the Research

After you have considered why research is important and gained an understanding of the different frameworks and designs used (section 1), and before you jump into your own study (Sections 3 to 5), it is important to prepare. Section 2 is divided into two different parts: finding what has already been done followed by methodological considerations.

Before you start your own study, go to the literature and see what has already been done on this topic. This is important well beyond making sure you are not 'reinventing the wheel'. It also ensures that you identify a gap in the literature that you can fill. Furthermore, knowledge of the existing literature is important to build up your background argument, get ideas on methodologies and be able to discuss and place your findings within the context of the larger body of existing evidence.

The literature review process can seem daunting at first, but follows a very structured approach and is often aided by software tools (Chapter 11). Once you are set up, understanding where and how to source the available literature follows (Chapter 12). There are many types of reviews, such as umbrella reviews, scoping reviews, rapid reviews and narrative reviews (Chapter 14) and more formal and less biased reviews such as Cochrane reviews and systematic reviews, including meta-analyses (Chapter 15). Once you have collected your literature, it needs to be appraised and critiqued (Chapter 13).

Once you have established what literature already exists but before you start filling the gap, there are some key methodological concepts to consider. Moral and ethical principles (Chapter 16) as well as cross-cultural considerations (Chapter 22) are paramount when designing research. How data will be collected and stored is more involved that it sounds (Chapter 17). Ensuring the data is reliable and valid is another key factor to consider (Chapter 18). Since you will only study a small number of participants from a large population, consideration should be given to sampling methods (Chapter 19) and sample size calculations (Chapter 20). Finally, an awareness of biases will strength the research output (Chapter 21).

11

Literature Review Process and Production Software

Bronwyn Beovich and Alexander Olaussen

LEARNING OUTCOMES

1. Be familiar with the steps to conduct a review of literature

2. Be aware of some software available to assist with completing a literature review

DEFINITION

'A literature review identifies, evaluates and synthesises the relevant literature within a particular field of research.'[1] As it is important for published reviews to be transparent and reproducible, the literature review process should be structured and follow consensus guidelines for reporting. A variety of software programs have been developed to aid many of the steps of a literature review.

INTRODUCTION

A literature review is a vital component of planning a research study on a topic to understand the existing literature and situate your research within it. There is a process to undertaking a literature review. A structured approach—as in clinical practice—ensures that vital components are not missed and helps manage an unfamiliar situation. The following 11 steps will guide you through the literature review process. This structure/process can be used for any type of review such as umbrella reviews, scoping reviews, rapid reviews, narrative reviews (Chapter 14) or Cochrane reviews and systematic reviews (Chapter 15).

11 STEPS TO CONDUCT YOUR OWN LITERATURE REVIEW

1. Develop your answerable research question.
2. Use a framework to assist in the development of your literature search strategy.
   - A commonly used mnemonic is PICO (Patient, problem or population; Intervention; Comparison, control or comparator; Outcome[s]) (see Chapter 6).
   - The mnemonic PCC (Patient, problem or population; Concept; Context) is recommended for scoping reviews.
3. Use online databases.
   - Search databases using both MeSH (Medical Subject Headings) terms and keywords (see Chapter 12).
   - Choose the databases to search that are relevant to your research question. Examples of databases that may be useful are:
     - Ovid MEDLINE (https://www.wolterskluwer.com/en/solutions/ovid/ovid-medline-901) and PubMed (https://pubmed.ncbi.nlm.nih.gov/), which contain a large number of paramedicine articles
     - CINAHL (Cumulative Index to Nursing and Allied Health Literature) (https://www.ebsco.com/products/research-databases/cinahl-complete),

which is also worth searching given the inclusion of allied health-specific literature.

4. Make an account with each database.
   - This enables you to save your searches as well as getting RSS feeds when new relevant articles are published.
5. Register the search if appropriate.
   - This is increasingly used for reviews to decrease duplication of research, minimise publication bias (where only studies with positive results are published) and increase transparency of the research process. The following two registries are available:
     - PROSPERO (https://www.crd.york.ac.uk/prospero/), which is used to register systematic reviews, rapid reviews and umbrella reviews

   - OSF (Open Science Framework) (https://osf.io), which may be used to register a variety of scientific projects, including scoping reviews.
6. Export references from the search into a reference manager.
   - There are many reference management software tools, of which EndNote is probably most widely used. However, there are other similar software programs (e.g. Mendeley, Zotero) with different features. Table 11.1 compares some of the available programs.
   - In choosing your software, consider cost, use of Google Docs versus Microsoft Word documents and what your supervisor/others in research team use (because you will share the reference library with each other).

TABLE 11.1 Features of Commonly Used Reference Management Software*

Software	Cost	Import File Formats	Cloud Storage	Word Processor Integration	Notes
EndNote[2]	Yes; may be free to use through institutional subscription Endnote basic (web version) free of charge	Ovid: yes PubMed: yes RIS: yes Other: yes	Increased risk of library corruption if using cloud storage (web version)	Microsoft Word: yes Microsoft Word online: no Google Docs: no	Support for > 6,000 citation styles
Mendeley[3]	Free	Ovid: no PubMed: yes RIS: yes Other: yes	Online storage free up to 2 GB; additional storage space may be purchased	Microsoft Word: yes Microsoft Word online: yes Google Docs: no	Support for > 8,000 citation styles
Paperpile[4]	Yes	Ovid: yes PubMed: yes RIS: yes Other: yes	Storage on Paperpile servers and some files stored locally within Chrome	Microsoft Word: under development Microsoft Word online: no Google Docs: yes	Support for > 8,000 citation styles; currently only on Google Chrome
RefWorks[5]	Institutional subscription	Ovid: yes PubMed: yes RIS: yes Other: yes	Yes	Microsoft Word: yes Microsoft Word online: yes Google Docs: yes	Support for > 13,000 citation styles
Zotero[6]	Free	Ovid: yes PubMed: yes RIS: yes Other: yes	Online storage free up to 300 MB; additional storage space may be purchased	Microsoft Word: yes Microsoft Word online: no Google Docs: yes	Support for > 9,000 citation styles

*Programs such as these often undergo modifications. Although the information above was deemed correct at the time of writing, we advise checking current program features prior to deciding on suitability for your project.

7. Remove duplicate articles.
   - This can generally be accomplished either in the reference manager program or a literature review management program such as Covidence (https://www.covidence.org/).
   - Be aware that if details of an article are recorded differently, the duplicate may not be identified.
   - Rather than optimising removal of duplicates at this stage of the search process, removal may be completed later in the process (e.g. during title/abstract screening).
8. Seek title/abstract screening.
   - This should be completed by two independent authors with reference to the inclusion and exclusion criteria of your literature review.
   - There is software available for this, such as Covidence (see Fig 11.1) which may be available free of charge via an institutional subscription.
   - Screening can be done on computer or smartphone.
   - Conflicts may be resolved by discussion and consensus, or by a third author.
9. Full text screening should also be undertaken by two independent authors, with conflicts resolved by consensus, or by a third author.
   - Articles excluded at this stage require justification as to why they have been excluded.
10. Confirm the final set of articles to be included in the review.
   - The results of the above steps are recorded in a PRISMA (Preferred Reporting Items for Systematic Reviews and Meta-Analyses) flow diagram; an updated version was published in 2020 (see Fig 11.2).
   - Consider, if feasible to do so, reporting the number of records identified from each database or register searched (rather than the total number across all databases/registers).
   - If automation tools were used, indicate how many records were excluded by a human and how many were excluded by automation tools.
11. Lastly, appraise the literature.
   - This is particularly important for systematic reviews.
   - See Chapter 13 for more details on article appraisal and tools.

EXAMPLES OF SYSTEMATIC REVIEWS

- Abetz JW, Olaussen A, Jennings PA, Smit DV, Mitra B. Pre-hospital provider clinical judgement upon arrival to the emergency department: a systematic review and meta-analysis. Emergency Medicine Australasia. 2020;32(6):917–23.
- Alqudah Z, Nehme Z, Alrawashdeh A, Williams B, Oteir A, Smith K. Paediatric traumatic out-of-hospital cardiac arrest: a systematic review and meta-analysis. Resuscitation. 2020;149:65–73.
- Funder JL, Ross L, Ryan S. How effective are paramedics at interpreting ECGs in order to recognize STEMI? A systematic review. Australasian Journal of Paramedicine. 2020;17.
- Shannon B, Pang R, Jepson M, Williams C, Andrew N, Smith K, Bowles, KA. What is the prevalence of frequent attendance to emergency departments and what is the impact on emergency department utilisation? A systematic review and meta-analysis. Internal and Emergency Medicine. 2020;15(7):1303–16.

CONCLUSION

Literature reviews are a valuable way to enable the identification and synthesis (plus or minus appraisal) of the existing literature within a topic area. Similar to clinical

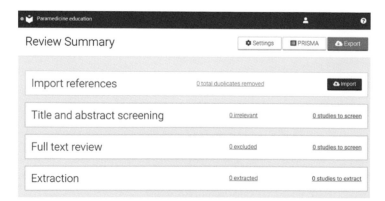

Figure 11.1 Covidence screenshot. (Source: Covidence. Online. Available from: https://www.covidence.org/.)

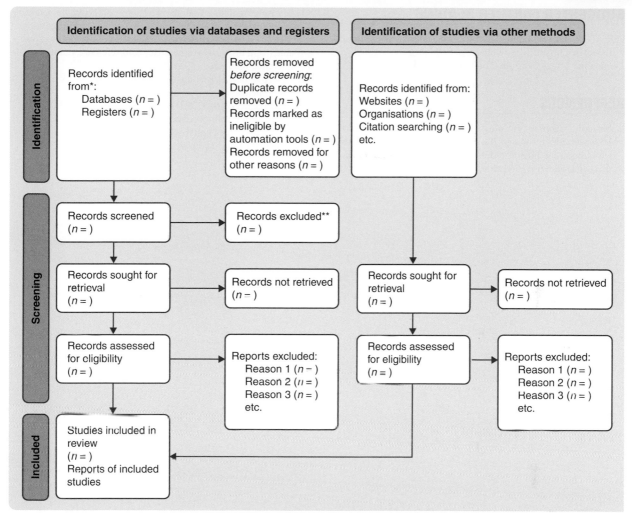

Figure 11.2 PRISMA 2020 flow diagram for new systematic reviews which included searches of databases, registers and other sources. (Source: Page MJ, Moher D, Bossuyt PM, Boutron I, Hoffmann TC, Mulrow CD, et al. PRISMA 2020 explanation and elaboration: updated guidance and exemplars for reporting systematic reviews. BMJ. 2021;372:n160.)

practice, the use of a systematic and comprehensive approach can help achieve an expertly accomplished task with a minimised chance of omitting important parts of the process. Although the highest evidence quality from a literature review is generally achieved with a systematic review (often accompanied by a meta-analysis), this type of research may not always be feasible or appropriate. Issues such as the amount of existing literature on a subject or time constraints may affect your choice of review. For assistance on which type of review best suits your requirements, please see Chapters 14 and 15. The use of appropriate software to assist with your review is encouraged.

REVIEW QUESTIONS

1. Think about an area within paramedic practice of which you would like more knowledge of the underpinning evidence. What PICO/PCC terms would assist you to identify relevant literature on the topic? What would be your answerable question?
2. Which referencing software program do you believe suits your research the most? Which factors would you consider in making your choice?

SUGGESTED FURTHER READING

EQUATOR (Enhancing the QUAlity and Transparency Of health Research): https://www.equator-network.org/

The Joanna Briggs Institute (JBI): https://jbi.global

REFERENCES

1. Monash University. Introduction to literature reviews. Learn HQ, Monash University. 2021. Online. Available from: https://www.monash.edu/rlo/graduate-research-writing/write-the-thesis/introduction-literature-reviews.

2. Clarivate Analytics. Endnote: For users. 2021. Online. Available from: https://clarivate.libguides.com/endnote_training/users.

3. Mendeley. Mendeley Reference Manager. 2021. Online. Available from: https://www.mendeley.com/reference-management/reference-manager.

4. Paperpile LLC. Paperpile. 2021. Online. Available from: https://paperpile.com/.

5. ExLibris. RefWorks®. 2021. Online. Available from: https://exlibrisgroup.com/products/refworks-reference-management/.

6. Corporation for Digital Scholarship. Zotero. 2021. Online. Available from: https://www.zotero.org/.

12

Sourcing the Available Evidence (Primary, Secondary and Tertiary Evidence)

Cameron M. Gosling and Ross Iles

LEARNING OUTCOMES

1. Define primary, secondary and tertiary evidence
2. Describe the sources of evidence that may be used in health and paramedicine research
3. Apply search strategies to source primary, secondary and tertiary evidence

DEFINITIONS

- Primary evidence: Original evidence that has not been altered by a third party.
- Secondary evidence: Information about a primary source that has been modified in some manner.
- Tertiary evidence: A collection of primary and secondary sources.
- Peer-reviewed literature: Publications that have been reviewed by two or more peer experts prior to acceptance for publication.
- Grey literature: A range of documents sourced from non-commercial publishers.

INTRODUCTION

Understanding the types of evidence, where that evidence comes from and how it is applied is important for any paramedic or paramedicine student. A cornerstone of evidence-based practice (EBP) is the identification, evaluation and application of appropriate research findings to clinical situations. Chapter 3 outlines how EBP links to the formulation of clinical guidelines and how that ultimately changes practice. However, before suitable evidence can be evaluated, it must be sourced. Ultimately, the strength of any review of information relies on how well the existing literature has been searched and how well the information is combined or synthesised.[1]

Historically, all evidence searches were completed by hand and often relied on a network of researchers disseminating information through limited peer-reviewed publications. As the breadth and depth of research has increased, so too has the number of journals and the manner in which we access them. Electronic health literature databases, such as MEDLINE, Cumulative Index to Nursing and Allied Health Literature (CINHAL), Scopus or Google Scholar are all examples that provide an easily accessible index of peer-reviewed health publications.

The rise in primary evidence is potentially the easiest source for paramedicine researchers and students to gather. This information represents new, original thoughts, discoveries or ideas. Primary evidence is the first presentation of results or events, through various media. This might include peer-reviewed journal publications, published conference abstracts or oral/poster conference presentations. Primary evidence may be robust, use sound scientific or experimental methods, and be evaluated through a peer-reviewed process. Or it may be anecdotal, based on casual observation rather than scientific evidence and not have been subjected to rigorous evaluation, such as vaccination misinformation.

Secondary evidence is information about one or more primary sources that has been modified. Such sources may describe, interpret, analyse and evaluate the primary source of information and provide a commentary about that evidence, such as a review of primary sources on a single topic. Some secondary sources use a rigorous scientific method, such as a Cochrane Collaboration review.[2] Others may pass through less stringent editorial oversight, commonly observed in the general popular media. In the research context, knowledge synthesis reviews have been classified into 48 different types.[3] Commonly used examples in paramedicine include systematic, meta-analysis, narrative, scoping and rapid reviews. In the past decade, a method to enhance the quality of searches used by each of these review types has been reported.[4] The quality of secondary evidence information is only as good as the sources it covers. Therefore, it is essential to capture all relevant primary sources to provide a complete overview of the topic being reported on.

The final evidence type, tertiary, is most commonly found in materials that have been modified, collated and re-analysed in a secondary form, then compiled into a concise evidence format, such as this textbook. Paramedics are familiar with these, as this type of evidence forms the basis of most clinical practice guidelines.

SEARCH PROCESS

Any search of the literature, regardless of whether it is for a student assignment or a funded research project, needs to have a structured approach. Search mistakes often happen when evidence is gathered through convenience, rather than a systematic approach.

Regardless of whether it is a systematic review with a meta-analysis or a scoping review to see what is out there, the starting point should be the creation of an answerable research question. The development of the question is enhanced when we use a format framework such as the PICO (Population, Intervention, Comparison and Outcome) approach (see Chapter 6 for more details).[5] Other approaches include SPIDER (Sample, Phenomenon of Interest, Design, Evaluation, Research type) often used for qualitative evidence synthesis,[6] or SPICE (Setting/Perspective (or Population)/Intervention/Comparison/Evaluation) used to evaluate outcomes of a specific intervention.[7] Knowing the types of evidence you are looking for can help to shape the question and guide the search.

It is important to plan an approach to ensure complete information is captured about our research question. Search strategy plans should be established for all research projects and be modified based on the type of review conducted. Your local university library should have guides on how to conduct effective evidence searches. Lately, researchers are disseminating their protocols through peer-reviewed publications and review registers such as the Cochrane Collaboration, Joanna Briggs Institute (JBI) and Prospero International Prospective Register of Systematic

Reviews. Some examples from the field of paramedicine include Reay and colleagues' systematic review protocol on transition in care[8] and Evans and colleagues' scoping review protocol on advanced clinical practice evidence[9].

A key part of any plan is to confirm that the search strategy will yield the required results. Recently, two paramedicine-specific search filters have been developed.[10] These filters have been optimised for sensitivity and specificity, meaning they include articles related to paramedicine when it should (true positive) and rules them out (true negative) when they are not relevant. Utilising these paramedicine-specific search strategies, an investigator can test and further refine the search to optimise output that will help to answer the research question.

Three further search strategies are important for evidence gathering, including grey literature, forwards and backwards searches. Depending on the topic, some public health information may only be available in the grey literature space.[10] For example, current paramedicine practice approaches to infectious respiratory diseases such as SARS or COVID may only be available through practice guidelines or clinical work instructions. Traditional literature searches may overlook these key documents. Grey literature can be harder to identify, as they may include sources such as government reports, theses and dissertations, conferences and proceedings, clinical trials and guidelines registers, and archived websites.[11] As this process can be time consuming, grey literature searches should be confined to information most relevant to your research question.

Forwards and backwards searches occur once literature has been included in the final sample of papers to review. This is a process specifically searching before and after an included article. Backwards searching is a process by which the reference list of an included article (those that came before the article) is scanned for relevant research not currently included in the search yield. A forward strategy is to review all prospective papers that have referenced the included article (those that came after), not yet included in your original search output.

CONCLUSION

The information we collect on a topic is only as good as the strategy we use to collect that evidence. A plethora of information is available to the paramedic. Sourcing evidence is about ensuring you have gathered all the relevant information, regardless of the type of evidence. The researcher then determines which of the sources collected are the best to use to answer their question. To accomplish this task, a critical appraisal of the collected information is required. Approaches to appraising the literature are presented in Chapter 13.

REVIEW QUESTIONS

1. What is the difference between primary, secondary and tertiary evidence and when would you use the different types?
2. What sources of evidence have you used and what are the benefits and drawbacks of the different sources?
3. What is meant by grey literature, forwards and backwards searches?

SUGGESTED FURTHER READING

Higgins JPT, Thomas J, Chandler J, Cumpston M, Li T, Page MJ, Welch VA, editors. Cochrane Handbook for Systematic Reviews of Interventions version 6.2 (updated February 2021). Cochrane, 2021. Online. Available from: https://training.cochrane.org/handbook.

Jordan Z, Lockwood C, Aromataris E, Munn Z. The updated JBI model for evidence-based healthcare. The Joanna Briggs Institute. 2016. Online. Available from https://jbi.global/jbi-model-of-EBHC.

Olaussen A, Semple W, Oteir A, Todd P, Williams B. Paramedic literature search filters: optimised for clinicians and academics. BMC medical informatics and decision making. 2017 Dec;17(1):1–6.

REFERENCES

1. Neilson CJ. Adoption of peer review of literature search strategies in knowledge synthesis from 2009 to 2018: an overview. Health Information and Libraries Journal. 2021;00:1–12. Online. Available: http://doi.org/10.1111/hir.12367.
2. Higgins JPT, Thomas J, Chandler J, Cumpston M, Li T, Page MJ, et al, editors. Cochrane Handbook for Systematic Reviews of Interventions version 6.2 (updated February 2021). Cochrane, 2021. Online. Available: http://www.training.cochrane.org/handbook.
3. Sutton A, Clowes M, Preston L, Booth A. Meeting the review family: exploring review types and associated information retrieval requirements. Health Information and Libraries Journal. 2019;36(3):202–22. Online. Available: http://doi.org/10.1111/hir.12276.
4. McGowan J, Sampson M, Salzwedel DM, Cogo E, Foerster V, Lefebvre C. PRESS Peer Review of Electronic Search Strategies: 2015 Guideline Statement. Journal of Clinical Epidemiology. 2016;75:40–6. Online. Available: http://doi.org/10.1016/j.jclinepi.2016.01.021.
5. Richardson WS, Wilson MC, Nishikawa J, Hayward RSA. The well-built clinical question: a key to evidence-based decisions. ACP Journal Club. 1995;123:A12–13.
6. Cooke A, Smith D, Booth A. Beyond PICO: the SPIDER tool for qualitative evidence synthesis. Qualitative Health Research. 2012;22(10):1435–43. Online. Available: http://doi.org/10.1177/1049732312452938.
7. Booth A. Clear and present questions: formulating questions for evidence based practice, Library Hi Tech. 2006;24(3): 355–68. Online. Available: https://doi.org/10.1108/07378830610692127.
8. Reay G, Norris JM, Alix Hayden K, Abraham J, Yokom K, Nowell L et al. Transition in care from paramedics to emergency department nurses: a systematic review protocol. Systematic Reviews. 2017;6:260. Online. Available: http://doi.org/10.1186/s13643-017-0651-z.
9. Evans C, Poku B, Pearce R, Eldridge J, Hendrick P, Knaggs R et al. Characterising the evidence base for advanced clinical practice in the UK: a scoping review protocol. BMJ Open. 2020;10:e036192. Online. Available: http://doi.org/10.1136/bmjopen-2019–036192.
10. Olaussen A, Semple W, Oteir A. et al. Paramedic literature search filters: optimised for clinicians and academics. BMC Medical Informatics and Decision Making. 2017;17:146. Online. Available: http://doi.org/10.1186/s12911-017-0544-z.
11. Adams J, Hillier-Brown FC, Moore HJ, Lake AA, Araujo-Soares V, White M, et al. Searching and synthesising 'grey literature' and 'grey information' in public health: critical reflections on three case studies. Systematic Reviews. 2016;5:164. Online. Available: http://doi.org/10.1186/s13643-016-0337-y.

13

Appraising and Critiquing the Evidence from Anecdotal, Observational and Experimental Studies Relevant to Paramedic Clinical Practice

Ted Brown and Luke Robinson

LEARNING OUTCOMES

1. Describe what research evidence is and why it is relevant to paramedic clinical practice
2. Recognise hierarchies of research evidence
3. Identify anecdotal, observational and experimental types of evidence
4. Explain methods for appraising and critiquing anecdotal, observational and experimental types

of evidence relevant to paramedic clinical practice
5. Identify and apply a variety of critical appraisal tools for different kinds of paramedic clinical practice research evidence

INTRODUCTION

This chapter will explore topics related to the appraisal and critique of anecdotal, observational and experimental research evidence relevant to paramedic clinical practice. Specifically, the importance of research evidence and hierarchies of evidence for paramedicine will be considered. Methods for appraising and critiquing anecdotal, observational and experimental research evidence, as well as specific types of critical appraisal tools, will then be discussed.

RESEARCH EVIDENCE AND ITS RELEVANCE TO PARAMEDIC PRACTICE

Research evidence is discipline knowledge, expert opinion, qualitative findings or experimental results that are collected in a systematic and replicable way to ascertain facts, trends and conclusions. Research evidence can be based on quantitative, qualitative or mixed methods study results. It provides the basis for all treatment and care protocols provided by medical, nursing and allied health professions, including paramedicine.[1]

Research evidence about specific clinical practices and procedures establishes which ones are efficacious or ineffective, cost-effective or expensive, and safe or harmful in the treatment of patients. Healthcare services and interventions based on best evidence have been found to improve patient health outcomes, reduce financial costs and increase patient satisfaction.[2]

HIERARCHIES OF RESEARCH EVIDENCE

Within research evidence, not all research designs are viewed as being equal. There is a definite research pyramid or hierarchy with some research designs being relegated to the bottom, middle and top of the level of evidence (LOE) tier.[3] The bottom of the research hierarchy includes single expert opinion, expert consensus, case series, pre-test/post-test, animal research/laboratory studies, observational-descriptive studies and anecdotal evidence. The middle of the hierarchy includes cohort, cross-sectional, case-control and quasi-experimental research designs.[4] The top of the research pyramid includes experimental designs, critically appraised topics, randomised controlled trials (RCTs), systematic reviews, meta-analyses and meta-syntheses.[5]

There are several well-recognised hierarchies of evidence or taxonomies that can be applied to rank the strength of the research evidence.[6] These include the Oxford Centre for Evidence-Based Medicine: Levels of Evidence (OCEBM-LOE), National Health and Medical Research Council Levels of Evidence (NHMRC-LoE) and the Joanna Briggs Institute Levels of Evidence (JBI-LOE).[7,8,9] All three LOE hierarchies also include levels of evidence for various purposes and types of research questions that are best answered by different types of research investigations, including intervention, diagnostic accuracy, effectiveness, diagnosis, prognosis, aetiology/harm, therapy, prevention, economic evaluations (cost) and meaningfulness. The OCEBM-LOE, NHMRC-LOE and JBI-LOE all focus on quantitative-based research evidence.

When considering qualitative research, Daly and colleagues have proposed a hierarchy that presents four levels of evidence: Level I Generalisable studies; Level II Conceptual studies; Level III Descriptive studies; and Level IV Single case studies).[10] The emphasis with this hierarchy is the ability of the research to provide evidence for use in practice or policy.

ANECDOTAL, OBSERVATIONAL AND EXPERIMENTAL EVIDENCE

There are several types of evidence, including anecdotal, observational and experimental. Anecdotal evidence depends mainly on personal experience and is typically collected in a casual, informal way (see Chapter 12 for more details on sourcing evidence).[11] Since personal involvement is the primary basis for anecdotal evidence, it is almost impossible to replicate and hence cannot be validated independently by other researchers or health professionals. When individuals believe their thoughts and ideas with certainty, they usually only turn to information that reinforces their views. This is referred to as 'predisposition' in the process of data, evidence and news retrieval.[12] People encounter anecdotal evidence from a variety of sources in their daily life including work colleagues, mentors, neighbours, friends, classmates, family members and social media.[13]

A second type of evidence is observational evidence. A step up from anecdotal evidence, the investigator scrutinises participants in their daily environments without them experiencing any form of intervention.[14] Observational studies can indicate if there are associations between two or more variables, but do not include control groups. Furthermore, observational research studies frequently guide the way forward in research as associations between variables can provide the basis on which research questions and

hypotheses can be investigated in the future in controlled experimental conditions.[15] Likewise, observational studies can assist investigators to be aware of what occurs in real-life daily situations and can be a form of data collection from standard practice.[16] Case-control and cohort study designs are two examples of observational studies. The findings of observational studies are often open to criticism by their nature and are often prone to confounding biases.[15]

Experimental evidence is generated by studies where one or more variables are manipulated or controlled by the researchers.[17] Typically, experimental studies are randomised with individuals randomly assigned to one of two or more participant groups. Usually, one group of study participants are assigned to a control or placebo group and the other group is allocated to an intervention group.[18] The researchers then compare the outcomes of the two groups, and any dissimilarities between the groups can be ascribed to the intervention. This allows causal inferences to be made about the variables being studied. Experimental evidence is often generated by RCTs where the findings are considered reliable since little is left to chance, and they are less prone to bias. It should be noted that generating experimental evidence is costly and time-consuming.[19]

METHODS FOR APPRAISING AND CRITIQUING RESEARCH EVIDENCE

Once anecdotal, observational and experimental evidence has been generated and then reported, it can be appraised and critiqued for its reliability, rigour, truthfulness, merits, limitations, potential biases, exposure to potential contaminating factors, implications and consequences.[20] The evidence-based process has several identified steps, and one of them is critically appraising the evidence. A critical review should be objective and impartial and present both the strengths and limitations of a study.[21]

When conducting a critical appraisal of a source of evidence, three basic questions need to be answered.
1. Is it worth looking at the results?
2. What are the results?
3. Are the results relevant for my patients?

This can be performed in a non-structured approach (e.g. critically appraise the evidence as it is read) or a structured approach (e.g. using a critical appraisal tool). The benefits and limitations of using each approach are presented in Table 13.1.

CRITICAL APPRAISAL TOOLS AND REPORTING GUIDELINES

Critical appraisal tools (CATs), also referred to as critical appraisal checklists, instruments or scales, provide a structured approach to completing analytical evaluations of the quality of a piece of evidence, with a focus on the methods that have been applied to minimise potential biases.[22] As these factors have the potential to influence results, and in turn, how they are interpreted, this information is essential to determine whether they can be believed and transferred appropriately into other environments such as policy, future research, education or clinical practice.[23] Therefore, choosing the most appropriate CAT is an essential component of evidence-based practice when completing a structured appraisal. Several CATs exist that can be used to assess the strengths and weaknesses of published studies. Table 13.2 presents several CATs that consider various study designs used when completing a structured appraisal of available evidence.

TABLE 13.1 Benefits and Limitations of Using Structured- and Non-Structured Appraisal Methods

	Non-Structured Appraisal	Structured Appraisal
Benefits	• Quick • Useful when you are working in a clinical setting • Useful when you need to read a large amount of evidence in a short period to determine best practice	• Involves a systematic and consistent approach • Can be used to determine an overall score of the quality of research • Can be replicated by other clinicians and researchers
Limitations	• Does not involve a systematic and consistent approach • Subjective appraisal of evidence	• Timely • Required to select the most appropriate CAT for the selected evidence

TABLE 13.2 Commonly Used Critical Appraisal Tools

Critical Appraisal Tool(s)	Authors	Appropriate for	Summary	Major Concepts
Critical Appraisal Skills Programme (CASP) checklists https://casp-uk.net/casp-tools-checklists/	CASP, Oxford, United Kingdom	Systematic reviews, RCTs, cohort studies, diagnostic studies, case-control studies, economic evaluation, clinical prediction rule, qualitative studies	Eight CASP checklists have been published and aim to allow students, researchers and practitioners to systematically assess the trustworthiness, relevance and results of published papers. Each checklist has between 10 and 12 items that are scored using 'Yes', 'No', or 'Can't tell' and provide prompts of important issues to consider alongside the questions. The checklists prompt reviewers to make comments to each item and complete an appraisal summary. An overall score of quality score is not calculated when using the various checklists as it has not been proposed by the authors.	The checklists contain various items depending on the study design considered. For example, the CASP RCT appraisal checklist considers the following. 1. Did the study address a clearly focused research question? 2. Was the assignment of participants to interventions randomised? 3. Were all participants who entered the study accounted for at its conclusion? 4. Were the participants/investigators/people assessing and analysing outcomes 'blind' to the interventions given? 5. Were the study groups similar at the start of the RCTs? 6. Apart from the experimental intervention, did each study group receive the same level of care (that is, were they treated equally)?

TABLE 13.2   Commonly Used Critical Appraisal Tools—cont'd

Critical Appraisal Tool(s)	Authors	Appropriate for	Summary	Major Concepts
				7. Were the effects of intervention reported comprehensively?
				8. Was the precision of the estimate of the intervention or treatment effect reported?
				9. Do the benefits of the experimental intervention outweigh the harms and costs?
				10. Can the results be applied to your local population/in your context?
				11. Would the experimental intervention provide greater value to the people in your care than any of the existing interventions?
Joanna Briggs Institute (JBI) checklists https://jbi.global/critical-appraisal-tools	Joanna Briggs Institute, Adelaide, Australia	Systematic reviews, RCTs, cohort studies, diagnostic test accuracy studies, case-control studies, case series, prevalence studies, economic evaluation, quasi-experimental studies, text and opinion, qualitative studies	JBI critical appraisal checklists have been developed by the JBI and collaborators and approved by the JBI Scientific Committee following extensive peer review. Although designed for use in systematic reviews, JBI critical appraisal checklists can also be used when creating critically appraised topics in journal clubs and as an educational tool. Each checklist presents an instruction guide for reviewers on how to interpret the question. An overall score of quality score is not calculated when using the various checklists as it has not been proposed by the authors.	The various checklists contain various items depending on the study design considered. For example, the JBI RCT appraisal checklist considers the following, 1. Was true randomisation used for assignment of participants to treatment groups? 2. Was allocation to treatment groups concealed? 3. Were treatment groups similar at the baseline? 4. Were participants blind to treatment assignment? 5. Were those delivering treatment blind to treatment assignment? 6. Were outcomes assessors blind to treatment assignment? 7. Were treatment groups treated identically other than the intervention of interest?

Continued

TABLE 13.2   Commonly Used Critical Appraisal Tools—cont'd

Critical Appraisal Tool(s)	Authors	Appropriate for	Summary	Major Concepts
				8. Was follow-up complete and if not, were differences between groups in terms of their follow-up adequately described and analysed? 9. Were participants analysed in the groups to which they were randomised? 10. Were outcomes measured in the same way for treatment groups? 11. Were outcomes measured in a reliable way? 12. Was appropriate statistical analysis used? 13. Was the trial design appropriate, and any deviations from the standard RCT design (individual randomisation, parallel groups) accounted for in the conduct and analysis of the trial?
Centre for Evidence-Based Medicine (CEBM) critical appraisal tools https://www.cebm.ox.ac.uk/resources/ebm-tools/critical-appraisal-tools	Centre for Evidence-Based Medicine, Nuffield Department of Primary Care Health Sciences, Oxford University, Oxford, United Kingdom	Systematic reviews, individual patient data (IPD) meta-analysis, RCTs, diagnostic studies, prognosis studies, qualitative studies	The CEBM critical appraisal tools were developed to help students, clinicians and researchers appraise the reliability, importance and applicability of clinical evidence. Each tool has a set of 'Yes', 'No' or 'Unclear' questions and prompts the reviewer to make comments for each section. An overall score of quality is not calculated when using the various checklists as it has not been proposed by the authors.	The various appraisal tools aim to answer four questions using various items depending on the study design that is under examination. 1. Does this study address a clearly focused question? 2. Did the study use valid methods to address this question? 3. Are the valid results of this study important? 4. Are these valid, important results applicable to my patient or population?

TABLE 13.2 Commonly Used Critical Appraisal Tools—cont'd

Critical Appraisal Tool(s)	Authors	Appropriate for	Summary	Major Concepts
Methodological Index for Non-randomised Studies (MINORS) https://onlineli-brary.wiley.com/doi/abs/10.1046/j.1445-2197.2003.02748.x	Slim K, Nini E, Forestier D, Kwiatkowski, F, Panis, Y, Chipponi, J	Non-randomised controlled trials, controlled before-and-after studies, interrupted time series studies, historically controlled studies, cohort studies, case-control studies, cross-sectional studies, case series	The MINORS contains 12 methodological points. The first eight apply to both non-comparative and comparative studies, while the remaining four relate only to studies with two or more groups. Every item uses 'Not reported (0 point)', 'Reported but inadequate (1 point) or 'Reported and adequate (2 point)' to appraise the study.	1. A clearly stated aim 2. Inclusion of consecutive patients 3. Prospective collection of data 4. Endpoints appropriate to the aim of the study 5. Unbiased assessment of the study endpoint 6. Follow-up period appropriate to the aim of the study 7. Loss to follow-up less than 5% 8. Prospective calculation of the study size 9. An adequate control group 10. Contemporary groups 11. Baseline equivalence of groups 12. Adequate statistical analyses
PEDro Scale, https://pedro.org.au/english/resources/pedro-scale/	The PEDro Partnership, Institute for Musculoskeletal Health, The University of Sydney and Sydney Local Health District, Sydney, Australia	RCTs	The PEDro scale was developed by the Physiotherapy Evidence Database to determine the quality of clinical trials. It consists of a checklist of 10 scored yes-or-no questions pertaining to the internal validity and the statistical information provided. Items are scored as either present (1) or absent (0) and a score out of 10 is obtained by summation.	1. Eligibility criteria were specified. 2. Subjects were randomly allocated to groups. 3. Allocation was concealed. 4. The groups were similar at baseline regarding the most important prognostic indicators. 5. There was blinding of all subjects. 6. There was blinding of all therapists who administered the therapy. 7. There was blinding of all assessors who measured at least one key outcome. 8. Measures of at least one key outcome were obtained from more than 85% of the subjects initially allocated to groups.

Continued

TABLE 13.2   Commonly Used Critical Appraisal Tools—cont'd

Critical Appraisal Tool(s)	Authors	Appropriate for	Summary	Major Concepts
				9. All subjects for whom outcome measures were available received the treatment or control condition as allocated or, where this was not the case, data for at least one key outcome was analysed by 'intention to treat'.
				10. The results of between-group statistical comparisons are reported for at least one key outcome.
				11. The study provides both point measures and measures of variability for at least one key outcome.

TABLE 13.3   Reporting Guidelines for Common Study Designs

Design	Reporting Guidelines
Systematic reviews and meta-analyses	Preferred Reporting Items for Systematic Reviews and Meta-Analyses (PRISMA statement; http://www.prisma-statement.org/)
Randomised trials	Consolidated Standards of Reporting Trials (CONSORT statement; http://www.consort-statement.org/)
Observational studies	STrengthening the Reporting of OBservational studies in Epidemiology (STROBE statement; https://www.strobe-statement.org/index.php?id=strobe-home)
Case reports	Consensus-based Clinical Case Reporting Guidelines (CARE guidelines; https://www.care-statement.org)
Qualitative research	COnsolidated criteria for REporting Qualitative research (COREQ; http://cdn.elsevier.com/promis_misc/ISSM_COREQ_Checklist.pdf)

While designed as a structured tool for researchers to use while writing manuscripts, reporting guidelines can be used to identify missing information the authors should have included. An online resource for reporting guidelines for many critical review guidelines is available at Enhancing the QUAlity and Transparency Of health Research (EQUATOR network; https://www.equator-network.org/).

Table 13.3 presents a summary of reporting guidelines for common study designs.

When appraising a randomised trial, for example, the Consolidated Standards of Reporting Trials (CONSORT) statement, which considers 25 items that should be reported (i.e. nature of randomisation method, blinding method etc.) could be used to identify omitted information or potential biases.

CASE STUDY

Low back pain (LBP) is a common reason why patients seek medical attention. Patients presenting with acute LBP may require transport to the hospital for assessment because of pain and immobilisation. Following an increase in the number of patients reporting minimal improvements from pharmacological interventions (e.g. opioids) taken prior to hospital arrival, an investigation into other interventions for LBP was undertaken. This poses a clinical issue relevant to paramedics.

A search of the literature for non-pharmacological pain management interventions for LBP during emergency transport resulted in the identification of an RCT titled 'Transcutaneous electrical nerve stimulation (TENS) reduces low back pain during emergency transport'.[24] The study aimed to investigate the effectiveness of paramedic-administered TENS in patients with acute LBP during emergency transport.

To assess the methodological quality of the RCT, a design in the top tier of the evidence hierarchy, the PEDro Scale (see Table 13.2), was applied and found the following.

- Eligibility criteria: Yes
- Random allocation: Yes
- Concealed allocation: Yes
- Baseline comparability: Yes
- Blind subjects: Yes
- Blind therapists: No
- Blind assessors: Yes
- Adequate follow-up: Yes
- Intention-to-treat analysis: No
- Between-group comparisons: Yes
- Point estimates and variability: Yes.
- Total score: 8/10 (Note: Eligibility criteria item does not contribute to total score.)

While some authors report that total PEDro scores of 0–3 are considered 'poor', 4–5 'fair', 6–8 'good' and 9–10 'excellent', it is important to note that these classifications have not been validated.[25] Furthermore, PEDro scores indicate that this is an appraisal of the study's methodological quality and not its findings and conclusions.

Therefore, based on a score of 8/10, this study is considered to be a fairly high-quality RCT and that the results achieved should be appraised and considered for use in practice. In this article, the authors found a significant (< 0.001) pain reduction for those exposed to the TENS intervention, whereas pain scores remained unchanged in the control group.

Based on the quality of the methodology (using the PEDro Scale), an appropriate number of participants in each group to ensure adequate power, and the findings (a significant reduction in pain scores), an argument for the use of TENS during transport for patients with LBP could be made.

In addition to the study above, a systematic review titled 'Transcutaneous electrical nerve stimulation for relieving acute pain in the prehospital setting: a systematic review and meta-analysis of RCTs' was retrieved as part of the literature.[26] To appraise the methodological quality of this investigation, the Critical Appraisal Skills Programme (CASP) Systematic Review checklist was used.

CONCLUSION

The ability to locate, appraise and critique empirical evidence relevant to clinical practice is an important skill required by many health professionals. In order to successfully appraise and critique anecdotal, observational and experimental types of evidence to ensure that paramedics are providing evidence-based interventions, it is essential to have a sound knowledge of study design principles, evidence hierarchies, and methods to appraise and critique available evidence. This chapter has provided an overview of these important evidence-based practice considerations and also provided a case study to illustrate how they can be used in clinical practice to guide treatment and policy.

REVIEW QUESTIONS

1. In the hierarchy of research evidence, what are two examples of top-level evidence?
2. What are three types of research evidence?
3. Describe the features of experimental research evidence.
4. What are the three questions that can be used to help guide a critical appraisal of a source of evidence?
5. What critical appraisal tools can be considered when appraising a randomised controlled trial?

REFERENCES

1. Simpson PM, Bendall JC, Patterson J, Middleton PM. Beliefs and expectations of paramedics towards evidence-based practice and research. International Journal of Evidence-Based Healthcare. 2012;10(3):197–203.

2. Lang ES, Spaite DW, Oliver ZJ, Gotschall CS, Swor RA, Dawson DE, et al. A national model for developing, implementing, and evaluating evidence-based guidelines for prehospital care. Academic Emergency Medicine. 2012;19(2):201–9.

3. Burns PB, Rohrich RJ, Chung KC. The levels of evidence and their role in evidence-based medicine. Plastic and Reconstructive Surgery. 2011;128(1):305–10.

4. Murad MH, Asi N, Alsawas M, Alahdab F. New evidence pyramid. BMJ Evidence-Based Medicine. 2016;21(4):125–7.

5. Ho PM, Peterson PN, Masoudi FA. Evaluating the evidence: is there a rigid hierarchy? Circulation. 2008;118(16):1675–84.

6. Long HA, French DP, Brooks JM. Optimising the value of the critical appraisal skills programme (CASP) tool for quality appraisal in qualitative evidence synthesis. Research Methods in Medicine & Health Sciences. 2020;1(1):31–42.

7. OCEBM Levels of Evidence Working Group. The Oxford 2011 levels of evidence. Oxford Centre for Evidence-Based Medicine. Online. Available: http://www cebm net/index aspx? o= 5653. 2011.

8. Merlin T, Weston A, Tooher R, Middleton P, Salisbury J, Coleman K. NHMRC levels of evidence and grades for recommendations for developers of guidelines. National Health and Medical Research Council (NHRMC) Canberra, ACT: Australian Government. 2009.

9. Joanna Briggs Institute. The Joanna Briggs Institute Levels of Evidence and Grades of Recommendation Working Party. Australia: Joanna Briggs Institute. 2014.

10. Daly J, Willis K, Small R, Green J, Welch N, Kealy M, et al. A hierarchy of evidence for assessing qualitative health research. Journal of Clinical Epidemiology. 2006;60(1):43–9.

11. Limb CJ. The need for evidence in an anecdotal world. Trends in Amplification. 2011;15(1):3–4.

12. Hornikx J. Combining anecdotal and statistical evidence in real-life discourse: comprehension and persuasiveness. Discourse Processes. 2018;55(3):324–36.

13. Alfred M, Jack S. Experts and anecdotes: the role of 'anecdotal evidence' in public scientific controversies. Science, Technology, & Human Values. 2009;34(5):654–77.

14. O'Neil M, Berkman N, Hartling L, Chang S, Anderson J, Motu'apuaka M, et al. Observational evidence and strength of evidence domains: case examples. Rockville: Agency for Healthcare Research and Quality. 2014;3(1):35.

15. Tavazzi L. Observational research as a platform for evidence-based public health policies and learning health systems. European Heart Journal. 2017;38(24):1891–4.

16. Bosiesz JR, Stel VS, van Diepen M, Meuleman Y, Dekker FW, Zoccali C, et al. Evidence-based medicine—when observational studies are better than randomized controlled trials. Nephrology. 2020;25(10):737–43.

17. Garbuio M. Experimental evidence. In: Augier M, Teece DJ, editors. The Palgrave encyclopedia of strategic management. London: Palgrave Macmillan UK; 2016. p. 1–4.

18. Barstow B, Fazio L, Schunn C, Ashley K. Experimental evidence for diagramming benefits in science writing. Instructional Science. 2017;45(5):537–56.

19. Martin A, Mikolajczak G, Orr R. Does process matter? Experimental evidence on the effect of procedural fairness on citizens' evaluations of policy outcomes. International Political Science Review. 2020:19251212090887.

20. Ingham-Broomfield R. A nurses' guide to the critical reading of research. Australian Journal of Advanced Nursing. 2014;32(1):37–44.

21. Dale JC, Hallas D, Spratling R. Critiquing research evidence for use in practice: revisited. Journal of Pediatric Health Care. 2019;33(3):342–6.

22. National Health and Medical Research Council. How to use the evidence: assessment and application of scientific evidence. Canberra: NHMRC; 2000.

23. Katrak P, Bialocerkowski AE, Massy-Westropp N, Kumar S, Grimmer KA. A systematic review of the content of critical appraisal tools. BMC Medical Research Methodology. 2004;4(1):22.

24. Bertalanffy A, Kober A, Bertalanffy P, Gustorff B, Gore O, Adel S, et al. Transcutaneous electrical nerve stimulation reduces acute low back pain during emergency transport. Academic Emergency Medicine. 2005;12(7):607–11.

25. Cashin AG, McAuley JH. Clinimetrics: Physiotherapy Evidence Database (PEDro) Scale. Journal of Physiotherapy. 2019;66(1):59.

26. Simpson PM, Fouche PF, Thomas RE, Bendall JC. Transcutaneous electrical nerve stimulation for relieving acute pain in the prehospital setting: a systematic review and meta-analysis of randomized-controlled trials. European Journal of Emergency Medicine. 2014;21(1):10–17.

14

Structured Reviews: Scoping, Rapid, Narrative and Umbrella Reviews

Paul Simpson and Robin Pap

LEARNING OUTCOMES

1. Differentiate between systematic reviews and other common types of reviews
2. Identify the methodologies, strengths and weaknesses of scoping, rapid, narrative and umbrella reviews
3. Select an appropriate review type based on set objectives

INTRODUCTION

Researchers often elect to undertake a review of the literature as an initial step in their research project, or as a self-contained project. A well conducted systematic review sits comfortably at the top of the 'hierarchy of evidence', and thus it can be easy for a researcher to feel drawn towards that review methodology as the 'gold standard' to aim for. This, of course, is true if the purpose of the review matches what a systematic review can offer. However, there are many purposes for which an alternative review method may be more appropriate. In an analysis of review typology conducted in 2009, Grant and Booth identified 14 types of literature review; these are detailed in Table 14.1.[1]

Given the many variants, one can easily become confused as to what type of review is most appropriate to select for a given project. Developing a familiarity with review typology and the strengths and weaknesses of each type will contribute towards informed decisions relating to choice of review methodology. A detailed description of all review types is beyond the scope of this chapter (though succinctly overviewed in Table 14.1); however, a closer examination of the more common variants is warranted. Systematic reviews, with or without meta-analyses, are discussed in Chapter 15 so will not be covered here. We will instead focus on scoping reviews, rapid reviews, narrative reviews and umbrella reviews.

COMMON REVIEW TYPES OTHER THAN THE SYSTEMATIC REVIEW

Scoping Reviews

Scoping reviews have become increasingly popular since their emergence in the late 1990s and are now underpinned by rigorous methodology.[2–4] There are six purposes for which a scoping review would be conducted:

1. identify the types of available evidence in a given field
2. clarify key concepts/definitions in the literature
3. examine how research is conducted on a certain topic or field
4. identify key characteristics or factors related to a concept
5. a precursor to a systematic review
6. identify and analyse knowledge gaps.[5, 6]

As can be seen by these purposes, the scoping review is not a less rigorous form of systematic review; it is a specific review type that demands a robust methodological approach to conduct and reporting.[3–5]

Applied Example

Birtill and colleagues scoped the concept of immersive simulation in undergraduate paramedicine education to clarify concepts and identify and analyse knowledge gaps as a precursor to informing an evolving suite of prospective research.[7] The scoping review approach was adopted due to the concept of immersive simulation being poorly defined and the need to scope the breadth and quality of existing literature.

TABLE 14.1   Main Review Types Characterised by Methods Used

| Label | Description | METHODS USED (SALSA) | | | |
		Search	Appraisal	Synthesis	Analysis
Critical review	Aims to demonstrate writer has extensively researched literature and critically evaluated its quality. Goes beyond mere description to include degree of analysis and conceptual innovation. Typically results in hypothesis or model	Seeks to identify most significant items in the field	No formal quality assessment. Attempts to evaluate according to contribution	Typically narrative, perhaps conceptual or chronological	Significant component: seeks to identify conceptual contribution to embody existing or derive new theory
Literature review	Generic term: published materials that provide examination of recent or current literature. Can cover wide range of subjects at various levels of completeness and comprehensiveness. May include research findings	May or may not include comprehensive searching	May or may not include quality assessment	Typically narrative	Analysis may be chronological, conceptual, thematic, etc.
Mapping review/ systematic map	Map out and categorise existing literature from which to commission further reviews and/or primary research by identifying gaps in research literature	Completeness of searching determined by time/scope constraints	No formal quality assessment	May be graphical and tabular	Characterises quantity and quality of literature, perhaps by study design and other key features. May identify need for primary or secondary research
Meta-analysis	Technique that statistically combines the results of quantitative studies to provide a more precise effect of the results	Aims for exhaustive, comprehensive searching. May use funnel plot to assess completeness	Quality assessment may determine inclusion/ exclusion and/or sensitivity analyses	Graphical and tabular with narrative commentary	Numerical analysis of measures of effect assuming absence of heterogeneity

Mixed studies review/ mixed methods review	Refers to any combination of methods where one significant component is a literature review (usually systematic). Within a review context it refers to a combination of review approaches; for example, combining quantitative with qualitative research or outcome with process studies	Requires either very sensitive search to retrieve all studies or separately conceived quantitative and qualitative strategies	Requires either a generic appraisal instrument or separate appraisal processes with corresponding checklists	Typically both components will be presented as narrative and in tables. May also employ graphical means of integrating quantitative and qualitative studies	Analysis may characterise both literatures and look for correlations between characteristics or use gap analysis to identify aspects absent in one literature but missing in the other
Overview	Generic term: summary of the [medical] literature that attempts to survey the literature and describe its characteristics	May or may not include comprehensive searching (depends whether systematic overview or not)	May or may not include quality assessment (depends whether systematic overview or not)	Synthesis depends on whether systematic or not. Typically narrative but may include tabular features	Analysis may be chronological, conceptual, thematic, etc.
Qualitative systematic review/ qualitative evidence synthesis	Method for integrating or comparing the findings from qualitative studies. It looks for 'themes' or 'constructs' that lie in or across individual qualitative studies	May employ selective or purposive sampling	Quality assessment typically used to mediate messages not for inclusion/ exclusion	Qualitative, narrative synthesis	Thematic analysis, may include conceptual models
Rapid review	Assessment of what is already known about a policy or practice issue, by using systematic review methods to search and critically appraise existing research	Completeness of searching determined by time constraints	Time-limited formal quality assessment	Typically narrative and tabular	Quantities of literature and overall quality/direction of effect of literature
Scoping review	Preliminary assessment of potential size and scope of available research literature. Aims to identify nature and extent of research evidence (usually including ongoing research)	Completeness of searching determined by time/scope constraints. May include research in progress	No formal quality assessment	Typically tabular with some narrative commentary	Characterises quantity and quality of literature, perhaps by study design and other key features. Attempts to specify a viable review

Continued

TABLE 14.1   **Main Review Types Characterised by Methods Used—cont'd**

| Label | Description | METHODS USED (SALSA) | | | |
		Search	Appraisal	Synthesis	Analysis
State-of-the-art review	Tend to address more current matters in contrast to other combined retrospective and current approaches. May offer new perspectives on issue or point out area for further research	Aims for comprehensive searching of current literature	No formal quality assessment	Typically narrative, may have tabular accompaniment	Current state of knowledge and priorities for future investigation and research
Systematic review	Seeks to systematically search for, appraise and synthesise research evidence, often adhering to guidelines on the conduct of a review	Aims for exhaustive, comprehensive searching	Quality assessment may determine inclusion/exclusion	Typically narrative with tabular accompaniment	What is known; recommendations for practice. What remains unknown; uncertainty around findings, recommendations for future research
Systematic search and review	Combines strengths of critical review with a comprehensive search process. Typically addresses broad questions to produce 'best evidence synthesis'	Aims for exhaustive, comprehensive searching	May or may not include quality assessment	Minimal narrative, tabular summary of studies	What is known; recommendations for practice. Limitations
Systematised review	Attempt to include elements of systematic review process while stopping short of systematic review. Typically conducted as postgraduate student assignment	May or may not include comprehensive searching	May or may not include quality assessment	Typically narrative with tabular accompaniment	What is known; uncertainty around findings; limitations of methodology
Umbrella review	Specifically refers to review compiling evidence from multiple reviews into one accessible and usable document. Focuses on broad condition or problem for which there are competing interventions and highlights reviews that address these interventions and their results	Identification of component reviews, but no search for primary studies	Quality assessment of studies within component reviews and/or of reviews themselves	Graphical and tabular with narrative commentary	What is known; recommendations for practice. What remains unknown; recommendations for future research

Source: Grant MJ, Booth A. A typology of reviews: an analysis of 14 review types and associated methodologies. Health Information and Libraries Journal. 2009;26(2):91–108.

Rapid Reviews

A rapid review is a simplified review methodology offering 'a streamlined approach to synthesising evidence in a timely manner—typically for the purpose of informing emergent decisions faced by decision makers in healthcare settings'.[8] While the systematic review is considered the 'gold standard', the time to produce it (between 6 and 24 months) and the complexity and volume of the final report create barriers to the efficient adoption of this knowledge in practice.[9, 10] A comparison between rapid and systematic reviews is illustrated in Table 14.2.

Applied Example

Pap and colleagues used a rapid review methodology to identify, appraise and summarise the best available evidence regarding pelvic circumferential compression devices and in doing so provided an evidence summary to inform an expert panel tasked to validate a related quality indicator used for the measurement of prehospital trauma care quality.[11] Given the large number of quality indicators that were being explored in the broader research project of which this study formed part, rapid reviews offered an efficient yet rigorous alternative to conducting multiple prolonged systematic reviews and enhanced the feasibility of the project.

Narrative Reviews

A narrative review, also often referred to as a literature review, is a review of the most important and critical aspects of a particular topic. In contrast to the systematic review with its rigorous methods, the narrative review is non-systematic, especially in terms of the search strategy but potentially also in terms of the specificity of the review question and the comprehensiveness of included studies. Despite these differences, which may be perceived as limitations, the narrative review is common in the medical literature and has a critical role in healthcare research.[12] The narrative review is superior to the systematic review in that it tends to address a topic in wider ways. Thus, a narrative review might be suitable as an initial exercise of a research project or to gain a broad understanding of an area of interest.

Applied Example

O'Meara and colleagues sought to inform the argument for the creation of an Australasian prehospital research agenda. They used a narrative review to draw on and discuss international experiences in achieving the same, and to identify methodologies on which an Australasian project could be based.[13] There was no need to engage in systematic quality appraisal of included articles and conduct an exhaustive literature search with systematic review rigour, and no specific question to be answered.

Umbrella Reviews

The increasing appetite for syntheses of existing research has led to a proliferation of review papers, particularly systematic reviews. In 2010 it was estimated that 11 new systematic reviews were published per day, resulting in an overwhelming volume of syntheses available for analysis and hopefully translation in to practice.[14] This proliferation spawned the emergency of the 'review of reviews', known now as the 'umbrella review'.

Whereas a standard review seeks to bring together relevant primary research papers in an all-encompassing review, the umbrella does the same but for existing reviews. It allows an examination of heterogeneity in outcomes across systematic reviews, and expedites the evidence synthesis process by not having to complete the full systematic review process on all studies included in the collection of systematic reviews.[15] While considered a relatively new

TABLE 14.2 General Comparison of Rapid Review versus Systematic Review Approaches[a]

	Rapid Review	Systematic Review
Timeframe[b]	≤ 5 weeks	6 months to 2 years
Question	Question specified a priori (may include broad PICOS)	Often a focused clinical question (focused PICOS)
Selection	Criterion-based: uniformly applied	Criterion-based
Appraisal	Rigorous: critical appraisal (SRs only)	Rigorous: critical appraisal
Synthesis	Descriptive summary/ categorisation of the data	Qualitative summary +/− meta-analysis
Inferences	Limited/cautious interpretation of the findings	Evidence-based

[a]Specific to the KTA [Knowledge to Action] program—other groups have experimented with other approaches of rapid review and will therefore have other differences.
[b]Primary difference; other potentially important differences are noted in the cells; PICOS = population, interventions, comparators, outcomes and study designs; SR = systematic review.
Source: Khangura S, Konnyu K, Cushman R, Grimshaw J, Moher D. Evidence summaries: the evolution of a rapid review approach. Systematic Reviews. 2012;1(1):1–9.

methodology, guidance frameworks for the conduct and reporting of umbrella reviews have been created and should be adhered to in order to promote quality, rigour and transparency.[14, 15] Umbrella reviews are uncommon in paramedicine, although opportunities increasingly exist.

Applied Example

De Freitas and colleagues applied umbrella review methodology to explore interventions aimed at improving patient flow in emergency departments in the United Kingdom.[16] Conscious of the number of systematic reviews on the same topic, their umbrella review encompassed 13 existing systematic reviews that covered 26 interventions.

CONCLUSION

This chapter provided a synopsis of some (not all) review types other than the systematic review. It is critical for researchers to carefully consider their a priori review objective(s) as this will best determine the most suitable review type. No review type is necessarily superior or inferior to another. However, poorly informed decisions around what type of review should be selected to answer a particular review question may lead to an inappropriate choice, and subsequently affect the quality of the review. It is usually advisable to consult library and information science workers when planning and conducting any type of review.

REVIEW QUESTIONS

1. As a paramedic who wishes to explore the literature on how quality in the context of paramedicine is defined, with the aim of mapping the breadth and scope of the current literature on the topic, what might be an appropriate review methodology? Explain your answer.
2. How does an author make sure they include all relevant paramedicine-related research articles in their review of the literature?

SUGGESTED FURTHER READING

Aromataris E, Munn Z, editors. JBI Manual for Evidence Synthesis. JBI; 2020. Online. Available: https://synthesismanual.jbi.global.

Noble H, Smith J. Reviewing the literature: choosing a review design. Evidence-Based Nursing. 2018;21:39–41.

REFERENCES

1. Grant MJ, Booth A. A typology of reviews: an analysis of 14 review types and associated methodologies. Health Information and Libraries Journal. 2009;26(2):91–108.
2. Pham MT, Rajić A Greig JD, Sargeant JM, Papadopoulos A, McEwen SA. A scoping review of scoping reviews: advancing the approach and enhancing the consistency. Research Synthesis Methods. 2014;5(4):371–85.
3. Peters MDJ, Godfrey C, McInerney P, Munn Z, Tricco AC, Khalil H. Chapter 11: Scoping reviews. In: Aromataris E, Munn Z, editors. JBI Manual for Evidence Synthesis. JBI; 2020. Online. Available: https://jbi-global-wiki.refined.site/space/MANUAL.
4. Tricco AC, Lillie E, Zarin W, O'Brien KK, Colquhoun H, Levac D, et al. PRISMA extension for scoping reviews (PRISMA-ScR): checklist and explanation. Annals of Internal Medicine. 2018;169(7):467–73.
5. Arksey H, O'Malley L. Scoping studies: towards a methodological framework. International Journal of Social Research Methodology. 2005;8(1):19–32.
6. Munn Z, Peters MD, Stern C, Tufanaru C, McArthur A, Aromataris E. Systematic review or scoping review? Guidance for authors when choosing between a systematic or scoping review approach. BMC Medical Research Methodology. 2018;18(1):1–7.
7. Birtill M, King J, Jones D, Thyer L, Pap R, Simpson P. The use of immersive simulation in paramedicine education: a scoping review. Interactive Learning Environments. 2021:1–16.
8. Khangura S, Konnyu K, Cushman R, Grimshaw J, Moher D. Evidence summaries: the evolution of a rapid review approach. Systematic Reviews. 2012;1(1):1–9.
9. Ganann R, Ciliska D, Thomas H. Expediting systematic reviews: methods and implications of rapid reviews. Implementation Science. 2010;5(1):1–10.
10. Munn Z, Lockwood C, Moola S. The development and use of evidence summaries for point of care information systems: a streamlined rapid review approach. World Views on Evidence-Based Nursing. 2015;12(3):131–8.
11. Pap R, McKeown R, Lockwood C, Stephenson M, Simpson P. Pelvic circumferential compression devices for prehospital management of suspected pelvic fractures: a rapid review and evidence summary for quality indicator evaluation. Scandinavian Journal of Trauma, Resuscitation and Emergency Medicine. 2020;28(1):1–13.
12. Bastian H, Glasziou P, Chalmers I. Seventy-five trials and eleven systematic reviews a day: how will we ever keep up? PLoS Med. 2010;7(9):e1000326.
13. O'Meara P, Maguire B, Jennings P, Simpson P. Building an Australasian paramedicine research agenda: a narrative review. Health Research Policy and Systems. 2015;13(1):1–5.
14. Aromataris E, Fernandez R, Godfrey CM, Holly C, Khalil H, Tungpunkom P. Summarizing systematic reviews: methodological development, conduct and reporting of an umbrella review approach. JBI Evidence Implementation. 2015;13(3):132–40.
15. Aromataris E, Fernandez R, Godfrey C, Holly C, Khalil H, Tungpunkom P. Chapter 10: Umbrella Reviews. In: Aromataris E, Z M, editors. JBI Manual for Evidence Synthesis. JBI; 2020. Online. Available: https://jbi-global-wiki.refined.site/space/MANUAL.
16. De Freitas L, Goodacre S, O'Hara R, Thokala P, Hariharan S. Interventions to improve patient flow in emergency departments: an umbrella review. Emergency Medicine Journal. 2018;35(10):626–37.

Cochrane Reviews and Systematic Reviews (Including Meta-Analyses and Meta-Synthesis)

Erin Smith and Paul A Jennings

LEARNING OUTCOMES

1. Discuss the role of systematic reviews and meta-analyses in making evidence-based decisions

2. Understand the characteristics of a systematic review

DEFINITIONS

A systematic review helps give an objective and transparent overview of all existing evidence surrounding a particular research question.

A meta-analysis is a statistical technique that enables data from more than one study to be combined and summarised as one overall dataset. This data summary is often presented as a forest plot or blobbogram.

INTRODUCTION

A systematic review is an important step in evidence-based practice (EBP). EBP is an approach to healthcare that integrates the best available research evidence with clinical expertise and patient values. It involves translating evidence into practice and ensuring that stakeholders, including health professionals, patients and family, are aware of and use research evidence to inform their health and healthcare decision-making.

Well-conducted systematic reviews are considered to be the most rigorous source of evidence, and as such sit at the top of the hierarchy of evidence, above randomised controlled trials. They identify, appraise and synthesise primary research papers using a clearly documented methodology which minimises bias. The clear documentation of the process and the decisions made allow the systematic review to be continually reproduced and updated.

CHARACTERISTICS OF A SYSTEMATIC REVIEW

The key characteristics of a systematic review include:[1]
- an answerable research question
- a transparent and reproducible search methodology that reduces the risk of bias
- clearly stated inclusion and exclusion criteria for studies
- an assessment of quality and validity of the findings of included studies
- a structured presentation and synthesis of the characteristics and findings of included studies.

COCHRANE REVIEWS

Cochrane is a network of international researchers and clinicians who share a mission to promote evidence-based decision-making through the production and curation of accessible systematic reviews and other synthesised research evidence. Cochrane publish five types of systematic reviews which have been rigorously prepared, including:
- reviews of effects of interventions
- reviews of diagnostic test accuracy
- reviews of prognosis
- reviews of methodology
- overviews of reviews.

Systematic reviews that follow the rigorous methods required by Cochrane and are accepted for publication in the Cochrane Database of Systematic Reviews in the

TABLE 15.1   Examples of How Systematic Reviews Can be Used

Use	Example
Recommendations and guidelines	Should paramedics refer patients to a community-based falls service?
Policy	Would it improve the health of our paramedics if we implemented annual physical fitness checks?
Performance measures	Does very early intervention by paramedics prior to arrival at hospital lead to improved clinical outcomes among sepsis patients?
Research agendas	What are the best methods for supporting paramedic mental health and wellbeing?
Patient care	What is the role of point-of-care ultrasound in prehospital critical care?
Patient decision-making	When should I call 000?

Cochrane Library (http://www.cochrane.org) are known as Cochrane reviews.[1]

WHAT ARE SYSTEMATIC REVIEWS USED FOR?

Systematic reviews are used to help make decisions to improve people's health.[2] Examples of how they can be used are shown in Table 15.1.

CONDUCTING A SYSTEMATIC REVIEW

The following tasks must be completed in order to conduct a systematic review.
1. Develop a clear, answerable research question, often utilising the PICO (Population, Intervention, Comparison and Outcome) format.
2. Pre-determine a transparent and reproducible search methodology.
3. Undertake a comprehensive search of appropriate databases for relevant data.
4. Extract data from identified studies using predefined inclusion and exclusion criteria.
5. Assess the quality and validity of the original research.

6. Present an overall synthesis of summary of results for all identified studies. This summary of results may be presented as a forest plot (or blobbogram), which is a graph that compares several clinical or scientific studies studying the same topic.[3]

HOW TO READ A FOREST PLOT

A forest plot will be presented as a series of lines and columns (see Fig 15.1). A description of each is provided below.[4]
- Column 1: Studies IDs
  - The first column on the forest plot shows the Study ID for the included studies.
- Column 2 and 3: Intervention and control groups
  - The next two columns show the intervention n/N and control group n/N; 'n' indicates the number of patients having the outcome of interest, while 'N' represents the total number of patients in that group.
- Column 4: Relative risk (fixed) 95% confidence interval (CI)
  - The next column visually displays the study results. The boxes show the effect estimates from the single studies, while the diamond shows the pooled result.
  - The horizontal lines through the boxes illustrate the length of the CI. The length of these lines represents the length of the CI. That gives you an estimate of how much uncertainty there is around that result—the shorter it is, the more confident we can be about the result.
  - The vertical line is the line of no effect, or the position at which there is no clear difference between the two groups.
  - If the outcome we are interested in is adverse (e.g. mortality), the results to the left of the vertical line favour the intervention over the control. That is, if result estimates are located to the left, it means that the outcome of interest (e.g. mortality) occurred less frequently in the intervention group than in the control group (ratio < 1).
  - If the outcome of interest is desirable (e.g. remission), the results to the right of the vertical line favour the treatment over the control. That is, if result estimates are located to the right, it means that the outcome of interest (e.g. remission) occurred more frequently in the intervention group than in the control group (ratio > 1).
  - If the diamond (the last possibility) touches the vertical line, the overall (combined) result is not statistically significant. It means that the overall outcome rate in the intervention group is much the same as in the control group. This is the case in this figure.

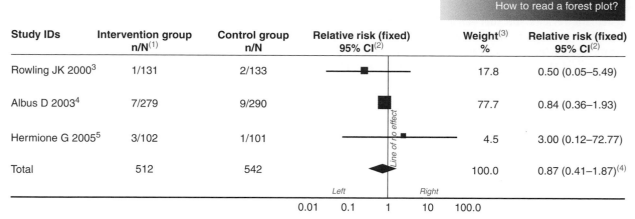

How to read a forest plot?

Study IDs	Intervention group n/N[1]	Control group n/N	Relative risk (fixed) 95% CI[2]	Weight[3] %	Relative risk (fixed) 95% CI[2]
Rowling JK 2000[3]	1/131	2/133		17.8	0.50 (0.05–5.49)
Albus D 2003[4]	7/279	9/290		77.7	0.84 (0.36–1.93)
Hermione G 2005[5]	3/102	1/101		4.5	3.00 (0.12–72.77)
Total	512	542		100.0	0.87 (0.41–1.87)[4]

Left   Right

0.01   0.1   1   10   100.0

Test for heterogeneity Chi-square = 0.79, df = 2, df = 2 , p = 0.67, I^2 = 0.0%[5]
Test for overall effect z = 0.35, p = 0.7[6]

(1) N = total number in group, n = number in group with the outcome.
(2) Outcome of interest in picture and in number. Fixed effect model used for meta-analysis.
(3) Influence of studies on overall meta-analysis.
(4) Overall effect.
(5) Heterogeneity (I^2) = 0%. So, we use fixed effect model.
(6) p value indicating level of statistical significance

Figure 15.1 Example of a forest plot. (Source: Cochrane UK. How to read a forest plot. 1 July 2016. Online. Available: https://uk.cochrane.org/news/how-read-forest-plot.)

• Note that this forest plot reports the relative risk; however, forest plots can report any measure of association (e.g. odds ratios, mean difference, prevalence).
• Column 5: Weight (%)
  • The weight (in %) indicates the influence an individual study has had on the pooled result. In general, the bigger the sample size and the narrower the CI, the higher the percentage weight, the larger the box and the more influence the study has on the pooled result.
• Column 6: Relative risk (fixed) 95% CI
  • The final column contains the same information as column 4, just in numerical format.
The p-value indicates the level of statistical significance. If the diamond shape does not touch the line of no effect, the difference found between the two groups was statistically significant. In that case, the p-value is < 0.05.

EXAMPLE

The following is an example of the role of systematic reviews in the evolution of a body of literature.[2]

Topic

Single-session critical incident debriefing for first responders.

Background

Critical incident debriefing (CID) has been used by emergency service organisations to help responders exposed to traumatic events. One type of approach involves single-session CID.

In 1995, an editorial identified five studies on the topic; none involved randomised comparisons.[5]

The first systematic review on the topic was published in 1998.[6] The same author conducted a more updated Cochrane review 4 years later, concluding that there was no evidence that single-session CID was useful treatment for the prevention of posttraumatic stress disorder (PTSD) after traumatic incidents.[7]

A more recent systematic review identified that recent evidence of the effectiveness of post-trauma CID is still lacking and remains inconclusive.[8]

Question

Based on the evolving evidence-base demonstrated in these reviews, what would you recommend to your organisation in regards to the use of CID?

CONCLUSION

Systematic reviews and meta-analyses play an important role when it comes to making healthcare decisions. They identify, evaluate and summarise the findings of all relevant individual studies on the same research question, thereby making the available evidence more accessible to decision-makers and consumers.

REVIEW QUESTIONS

1. What is the benefit of 'pooling' data from a number of primary studies to undertake a meta-analysis?
2. Systematic reviews can take a long time to complete, sometimes 2 years or more. In what ways may this impact our quest for rigorous evidence from which to assist with decision-making and policy development?
3. Consider an answerable research (PICO) question using the information provided in the example in this chapter.

SUGGESTED FURTHER READING

Gough D, Oliver S, Thomas J. An introduction to systematic reviews. 2nd ed. London: SAGE Publications; 2017.

SUGGESTED VIEWING

Cochrane. What are systematic reviews? 28 January 2016. Online. Available: https://www.youtube.com/watch?v= egJlW4vkb1Y.

REFERENCES

1. Higgins JP, Thomas J, editors. Cochrane handbook for systematic reviews of interventions version 6.2. Cochrane Training; 2021. Online. Available: http://www.training.cochrane.org/handbooks.
2. Elizabeth OC, Whitlock E, Spring, B. Introduction to systematic reviews. Evidence-based Behavioral Practice. Online. Available: https://ebbp.org/training/systematicreview.
3. Lewis S, Clarke M. Forest plots: trying to see the wood and the trees. BMJ. 2001;322(7300):1479–80.
4. Cochrane UK. How to read a forest plot. 1 July 2016. Online. Available: https://uk.cochrane.org/news/how-read-forest-plot.
5. Raphael B, Meldrum L, McFarlane, A. Does debriefing after psychological trauma work? BMJ. 1995;310:1479–80.
6. Rose S, Bisson J. Brief early psychological interventions following trauma: A systematic review of the literature. Journal of Traumatic Stress. 1998;11:697–710.
7. Rose S, Bisson J, Churchill R, Wessely S. Psychological debriefing for preventing post-traumatic stress disorder (PTSD). Cochrane Database of Systematic Reviews. 2002;(2):CD000560.
8. Anderson GS, Di Nota PM, Groll D, Carleton RN. Peer support and crisis-focused psychological interventions designed to mitigate post-traumatic stress injuries among public safety and frontline healthcare personnel: a systematic review. International Journal of Environmental Research and Public Health. 2020;17:7645. Online. Available: http://doi.org/10.3390/ijerph17207645.

16

Moral Principles and Ethical Considerations

David Reid

LEARNING OUTCOMES

1. Describe the difference between law and ethics
2. Identify the four principles of medical bioethics
3. Outline ethical challenges in the prehospital environment
4. Describe ethical governance and the content of a research ethics application

DEFINITIONS

- Bioethics: The study of ethical implications of medical, biological and environmental research.[1]
- Ethics: A field of moral philosophy dealing with the standards by which behaviour should be regulated.[2]
- Law: The principles and regulations emanating from a government and applicable to a people, whether in the form of legislation or of custom and policies recognised and enforced by judicial decision.[1]
- Morals: Principles or habits with respect to right or wrong conduct.[1]

INTRODUCTION

The paramedicine researcher has an obligation to protect their research participants from harm, and this is the primary goal of ethical considerations in research. While there is no single unified code for paramedicine research, the Australian Code for the Responsible Conduct of Research (the Code) is published by the National Health and Medical Research Council (NHMRC) and sets out the broad principles that characterise honest, ethical and conscientious research.[3] Their National Statement on Ethical Conduct in Human Research outlines the key principles

in relation to human research.[4] Other ethical codes of practice are published by higher education institutions, professional bodies such as the Australasian College of Paramedicine and the Paramedicine Board of Australia as part of their codes of conduct.[5,6] This chapter outlines the broad moral and ethical considerations applicable to paramedical science research.

ETHICS VERSUS LAW

In Australia the law is set at various levels of government including local, state and Commonwealth. Acts are passed by Parliament at state/territory and Commonwealth levels, and Regulations are subordinate to the Acts.[7] In addition to statutory law there exists a significant body of case (or common) law, developed by judges from civil and criminal trials. Many legal rules develop through judicial precedence, by which judges are bound by earlier decisions on the same point of law.[8] The law needs to be followed in any research project.

Ethics is underpinned by morality, and the view of morality (and hence ethics) will vary from person to person.[9] According to Kohlberg, an individual's morals are influenced by such factors as avoidance of punishment, development of individual viewpoints, interpersonal relationships, the social order, social versus individual rights and their own set of universal moral principles.[10] An individual's morals may change over their life span.[10]

There are three main ethical theories: consequentialist, deontological and virtuous. A consequential viewpoint holds that an act is considered morally 'right' based on the consequence of the act itself. If the act provides greatest good to the greatest number then the act is ethical.[11] Deontological ethics suggests that an act is ethical if it conforms to a set of rules, irrespective of its consequences.[11] Finally, virtuous ethics, the oldest of the three approaches, suggests that morally good actions will exemplify virtues and morally bad actions will be vices.[11] In paramedicine research, the researcher will be guided by their own morals as to the type of research, the limits of participant involvement and what constitutes 'ethical' research.

PRINCIPLES OF BIOETHICS

In practice, the paramedicine researcher, regardless of their own morals and ethical viewpoint as just outlined, is generally bound by the four principles of bioethics which are often embedded in research codes of practice.[12] The principles of bioethics place the research subject at the centre of research and provide a simple framework and reference point for ensuring research participant safety. The four principles of bioethics, outlined in Figure 16.1 are autonomy, non-maleficence, beneficence and justice.

PARAMEDICAL RESEARCH

Unlike many areas of research, prehospital care is characterised by unpredictability, urgency of care and an uncontrolled prehospital environment.[13] These characteristics make it challenging for the prehospital researcher to design research that fully satisfies all four biomedical ethical principles. Therefore, there may be trade-offs between the four principles to advance prehospital knowledge. The published literature has highlighted autonomy, exemplified through capacity and consent, as being a particularly challenging aspect of ethics in prehospital research.[13,14] Other ethical challenges identified in the prehospital environment include patient privacy, difficulty in follow-up, variability of practice, infrastructure complexity and cost, and adequately powering studies to ensure valid conclusions can be reached.[14]

ETHICAL GOVERNANCE AND ETHICS APPLICATIONS

Ethical considerations in paramedical research are separate to the laws and regulations published by government. Additionally, an ambulance service, professional representative body or university may publish research guidelines. The paramedic is expected to be conversant with all of these prior to commencing their research. The NHMRC outlines eight key principles of responsible research conduct

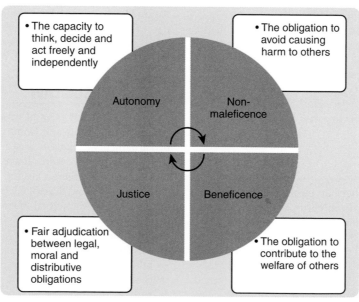

Figure 16.1 Principles of biomedical ethics. (Source: Beauchamp TL, Childress JF. Principles of biomedical ethics. 8th ed. New York, NY: Oxford University Press; 2019.)

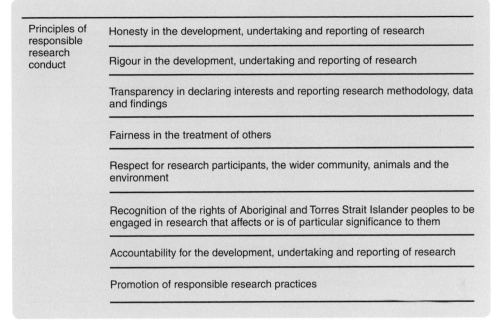

Principles of responsible research conduct	Honesty in the development, undertaking and reporting of research
	Rigour in the development, undertaking and reporting of research
	Transparency in declaring interests and reporting research methodology, data and findings
	Fairness in the treatment of others
	Respect for research participants, the wider community, animals and the environment
	Recognition of the rights of Aboriginal and Torres Strait Islander peoples to be engaged in research that affects or is of particular significance to them
	Accountability for the development, undertaking and reporting of research
	Promotion of responsible research practices

Figure 16.2 Principles of responsible research conduct. (Source: National Health and Medical Research Council. Australian code for the responsible conduct of research. Canberra: NHMRC; 2018.)

(see Fig 16.2). These principles underpin ethics applications which will be required as part of any formal research.

Paramedical research will require ethics approval, usually from a multidisciplinary research ethics committee. The role of these committees is to ensure that the ethical issues and welfare of research participants can be safely combined with the scientific aspects of a proposed research study.[15] Within ambulance services, these committees may be internally constituted or may be outsourced to a university research partner. Prior to commencing the data collection phase, the paramedicine researcher will find that ethics approval is required. Ethics approval is given after submission of an ethics approval form where the paramedicine researcher explains their research methodology and approach, and outlines their ethical considerations and how they will be addressed to promote research participant safety. Examples of information required, commensurate with the level of risk to the researcher and research participants, in an ethics application may include:[16]

- project title
- experience of researcher(s)
- scope, aims and objectives of the research
- research methodology
- participant recruitment process
- information letters and brochures
- consent form

- collection, use and management of research data (including storage and disposal)
- dissemination of research findings
- risk assessment
- legal considerations (e.g. privacy, records management).

When assessing an ethics application, a research ethics committee will examine issues such as the validity of the research, the welfare of research participants and whether dignity of research participants is respected (see Fig 16.3).[17]

After ethics approval is granted, paramedical researchers will find they are subject to regular ethics reports which, as well as outlining research progress, may require disclosure of:

- any changes to project methodology
- extensions to project timelines
- disclosure of adverse or unintended events
- confirmation of compliance with research project conditions and/or NHMRC codes.

SPECIAL POPULATIONS

In their National Statement on Ethical Conduct in Human Research, the NHMRC outlines key considerations in relation to special populations (see Fig 16.4) who may be involved in research.[4] These populations have been identified as being at greater risk of harm during research or at

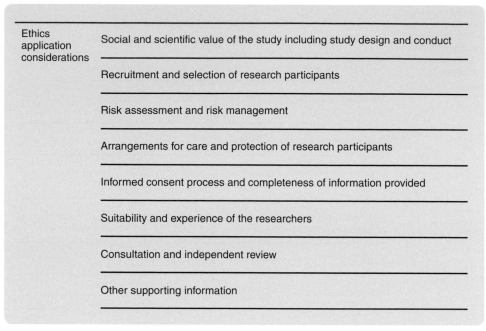

Ethics application considerations

Social and scientific value of the study including study design and conduct

Recruitment and selection of research participants

Risk assessment and risk management

Arrangements for care and protection of research participants

Informed consent process and completeness of information provided

Suitability and experience of the researchers

Consultation and independent review

Other supporting information

Figure 16.3 Research ethics application review. (Source: George AJT. Research ethics. Medicine. 2016; 44(10):615–8.)

Special populations

Pregnant women and the human fetus

Children and young people

People in dependent or unequal relationships

People highly dependent on medical care who may be unable to give consent

People with a cognitive impairment, an intellectual disability or a mental illness

People who may be involved in illegal activities

Aboriginal and Torres Strait Islander peoples

People in other countries

Figure 16.4 Special populations. (Source: National Health and Medical Research Council. National statement on ethical conduct in human research. Canberra: NHMRC; 2018.)

greater risk during the consent-to-research process, and therefore require specific ethical considerations. If the paramedicine researcher's study involves these populations, additional ethical safeguards will be required.

CONCLUSION

The paramedicine researcher has an ethical obligation to safeguard their research participants from harm. The Australian Code for the Responsible Conduct of Research outlines the broad principles that characterise ethical research. Ethics is separate to the law, and the paramedicine researcher is required to abide by both the law and any ethical considerations. The four principles of bioethics, although challenging in the prehospital environment, often underpin the responsibility on the paramedicine researcher. Prior to commencing data collection, the paramedicine researcher will be required to submit an ethics application to a research ethics committee, outlining their ethical considerations and how they will address them as part of the research. Following approval, the researcher will be required to provide ethics reports.

REVIEW QUESTIONS

1. Define ethics and outline the three main ethical viewpoints.
2. Describe the four principles of bioethics and outline the eight NHMRC principles of responsible research conduct.
3. What characteristics make the paramedicine research environment unique?
4. Define the role of a research ethics committee and identify which aspects of a research ethics application would be examined by them.
5. Provide four examples of special populations requiring particular ethical consideration.

SUGGESTED FURTHER READING

National Health and Medical Research Council: Australian Code for the Responsible Conduct of Research. Online. Available: https://www.nhmrc.gov.au/about-us/publications/australian-code-responsible-conduct-research-2018

National Health and Medical Research Council: National Statement on Ethical Conduct in Human Research. Online. Available: https://www.nhmrc.gov.au/about-us/publications/national-statement-ethical-conduct-human-research-2007-updated-2018

World Medical Association Declaration of Helsinki – Ethical Principles for Medical Research Involving Human Subjects.

Online. Available: https://www.wma.net/policies-post/wma-declaration-of-helsinki-ethical-principles-for-medical-research-involving-human-subjects/

REFERENCES

1. Macquarie Dictionary Online. 8th ed. Sydney: Pan Macmillan; 2020.
2. Jupp V. The SAGE dictionary of social research methods. London: SAGE Publications; 2006. Online. Available: http://www.123library.org/book_details/?id=377.
3. National Health and Medical Research Council. Australian code for the responsible conduct of research. Canberra: NHMRC; 2018.
4. National Health and Medical Research Council. National statement on ethical conduct in human research. Canberra: NHMRC; 2018.
5. Australasian College of Paramedicine. Governance. 2021. Online. Available: https://paramedics.org/governance.
6. Paramedicine Board Ahpra. Code of conduct. 2021. Online. Available: https://www.paramedicineboard.gov.au/Professional-standards/Codes-guidelines-and-policies/Code-of-conduct.aspx.
7. Clark D. Introduction to Australian public law. Sydney: LexisNexis Butterworths; 2016. Online. Available: http://public.eblib.com/choice/PublicFullRecord.aspx?p=6226429.
8. Harpwood V. Law and ethics in medicine. Medicine. 2020;48(10):664–6.
9. Charlton K, Franklin J, McNaughton R. Phenomenological study exploring ethics in prehospital research from the paramedic's perspective: experiences from the Paramedic-2 trial in a UK ambulance service. Emergency Medicine Journal. 2019;36(9):535–40.
10. Kohlberg L. Collected papers on moral development and moral education. Cambridge, Mass.: Harvard University; 1973.
11. Bench-Capon TJM. Ethical approaches and autonomous systems. Artificial Intelligence. 2020;281.
12. Beauchamp TL, Childress JF. Principles of biomedical ethics. 8th ed. New York, NY: Oxford University Press; 2019.
13. Armstrong S, Langlois A, Siriwardena N, Quinn T. Ethical considerations in prehospital ambulance based research: qualitative interview study of expert informants. BMC Medical Ethics. 2019;20(1):88.
14. Miskimins R, Pati S, Schreiber M. Barriers to clinical research in trauma. Transfusion. 2019;59(S1):846–53.
15. Snowden R. Principles of research ethics. Journal of Paramedic Practice. 2021;3(10):1.
16. Edith Cowan University. Applying for research ethics approval. 2021. Online. Available: https://intranet.ecu.edu.au/research/research-ethics-and-integrity/applying-for-research-ethics-approval.
17. George AJT. Research ethics. Medicine. 2016;44(10):615–8.

Data Collection and Storage

Emily Andrew and Ziad Nehme

LEARNING OUTCOMES

1. Understand the concept of research data management
2. Understand data collection in the setting of out-of-hospital research
3. Appropriately store, retain and dispose of research data

DEFINITIONS

Data management is a broad term that encompasses the appropriate collection, storage, retention and disposal of research data.[1,2] Effective data management:
1. ensures data integrity and quality
2. decreases the risk of loss or inappropriate use of data.

INTRODUCTION

The Australian Code for the Responsible Conduct of Research (2018) requires researchers to observe appropriate generation, collection, access, analysis, storage, retention and disposal of data and information.[1,2] As the foundation on which research hypotheses are evaluated, accurate data collection is arguably the most important step in the research process. Prior to data collection, a data management plan should be completed.

DATA COLLECTION

Research data may be either quantitative (measures of quantity) or qualitative (measures of 'types' or themes).[3] Quantitative out-of-hospital research data may be collected from a variety of sources. Examples include retrospective data from paramedic electronic patient care records, computer-aided dispatch records and clinical quality registries, as well as prospective data from surveys and project-specific data collection forms. Linkage of ambulance service data with hospital records is also becoming increasingly popular as it provides an indication of patient outcomes after paramedic handover at hospital. Further, linkage enables assessment of prehospital factors that may be associated with patient outcomes. Qualitative out-of-hospital research data may be collected from focus groups or interviews (e.g. with paramedics or ambulance service staff). Qualitative and quantitative research data may also be collected from published journal articles for systematic reviews and meta-analyses.

All data should be collected in accordance with an approved study protocol, and only those data that meet the purpose of the research should be collected. Collected data elements should be defined within a data dictionary.

DATA VERIFICATION

After data collection, data must undergo quality control, checks for accuracy and coding.[4] Data which are collected prospectively and/or specifically for research purposes are generally accepted to be more accurate than clinical data which are collected primarily as a health record. This is due predominantly to differing priorities in clinical and research settings.[5] In the case of paramedic patient care records, quality control and data coding is essential prior to analysis. Examples of quality control checks include assessing for missing data, duplicates and outliers, as well as ensuring consistency in data capture. Upon completion of data quality checks, quantitative and qualitative data are often coded into meaningful categories before analysis.

DATA STORAGE

All research data should be stored on computing systems that are secure and accessible only to those researchers who have received ethical approval for access. The security classification of the collected research data, which includes very sensitive (e.g. identifiable), sensitive (e.g. re-identifiable) and restricted (e.g. de-identified, aggregated) information, often determines the researcher's responsibility in regards to data access, storage, retention and disposal.[4] For example, access to very sensitive information should be strictly limited. Research data are rarely provided to a third party without ethical and ambulance service approval. However, if data is transferred between parties, transfer should occur via a secure electronic transmission platform. Backing up research data is recommended.

DATA RETENTION

Upon completion of a research project, researchers are responsible for securely archiving data and for destroying it after a specified time. It is generally accepted that the minimum period for data retention is 5 years from the date of publication, although many institutions recommend retaining data for 7 years. In the case of clinical trials, data should be retained for 15 years or more.[2]

Examples

Retrospective Data Collection with Data Linkage

In 2017, Australian researchers conducted a retrospective cohort study of patients with non-traumatic brain pathologies who had received rapid sequence intubation (RSI) from intensive care paramedics in Victoria.[6] Patients who were transported to one of seven Melbourne hospitals were included. Data were collected from the Ambulance Victoria clinical data warehouse which stores all data recorded within paramedic electronic patient care records. Extracted data elements included patient identifiers, pre-hospital interventions, time intervals, final assessment and vital signs. For patients who received RSI, data was linked with hospital outcomes, and patients with a hospital diagnosis related to a non-traumatic brain pathology were included in the final study. Following data collection, data verification and coding was undertaken.

Given that identifiable patient data was required to facilitate linkage with hospital records, the authors outlined several risk mitigation strategies within their study protocol to ensure patient confidentiality and data security. The research data will be archived until at least 2024.

Prospective Data Collection Using a Project-Specific Data Collection Form

An international group of researchers conducted a prospective observational study in four countries to observe hand hygiene compliance, glove behaviour and adherence to basic hygiene parameters in emergency medical service providers.[7] With ethical, ambulance service and participating paramedic approval, two researchers each completed 30 hours of ambulance observer shifts in each country. During their observations, the researchers completed a project-specific data collection form which included recording the use of hand rubbing, hand washing and gloves, as well as nail length and the wearing of rings and/or watches. The collected data did not contain identifying information. Data collection initially occurred on paper forms before entry into a statistical software for analysis. To prevent data entry errors, data elements were evaluated in relation to predefined expected values. Paper report forms were destroyed once electronic data had been checked for accuracy. Study data was stored securely on lead researcher's organisational network drive. The study was published in 2019 and data will remain archived until at least 2026.

CONCLUSION

Out-of-hospital research data may be collected from a variety of sources. As the basis upon which research hypotheses are evaluated or generated, it is important to ensure data accuracy. Data should be stored securely during the research process and archived for an appropriate period after the completion of the research project.

REVIEW QUESTIONS

1. Why is accurate research data collection important?
2. How should data be stored during and after completion of the research project?

SUGGESTED FURTHER READING

Lee LM, Gostin LO. Ethical collection, storage, and use of public health data: a proposal for a national privacy protection. JAMA. 2009 Jul 1;302(1):82–4. https://pubmed.ncbi.nlm.nih.gov/19567443/.

National Health and Medical Research Council. Australian code for the responsible conduct of research. Canberra: NHMRC; 2018.

The research data management and good research practice guidelines at your university.

REFERENCES

1. National Health and Medical Research Council. Australian code for the responsible conduct of research. Canberra: NHMRC; 2018.
2. National Health and Medical Research Council. Management of data and information in research: a guide supporting the Australian code for the responsible conduct of research. Canberra: NHMRC; 2019.
3. Shah A. Using data for improvement. BMJ. 2019;364:l189.
4. Monash Public Health and Preventive Medicine. A guide to good research practice. Melbourne, Australia: Monash University, 2020.
5. Weiskopf NG, Weng C. Methods and dimensions of electronic health record data quality assessment: enabling reuse for clinical research. Journal of the American Medical Informatics Association. 2013;20(1):144–51.
6. Fouche PF, Jennings PA, Smith K, Boyle M, Blecher G, Knott J, et al. Survival in out-of-hospital rapid sequence intubation of non-traumatic brain pathologies. Prehospital Emergency Care. 2017;21(6):700–8.
7. Vikke HS, Vittinghus S, Giebner M, Kolmos HJ, Smith K, Castrén M, et al. Compliance with hand hygiene in emergency medical services: an international observational study. Emergency Medicine Journal. 2019;36(3):171–5.

18

Reliability and Validity in Quantitative and Qualitative Research

Richard Armour and Brett Williams

LEARNING OUTCOMES

1. Define and explore the concept of reliability as it applies to quantitative and qualitative research
2. Define and explore the concept of validity as it applies to quantitative and qualitative research
3. Outline methods by which reliability and validity are assessed in published literature
4. Describe common threats to reliability and validity in both quantitative and qualitative research

INTRODUCTION

Both quantitative and qualitative research methodologies may be applied in paramedic research as we seek to understand not just the 'what' of paramedic practice, but also the 'why'. When conducting and reviewing both quantitative and qualitative research, though, it is critical that we are satisfied the research is both accurate and free from error so much as is feasibly possible. A careful, considered methodological approach will assist in achieving these goals, with particular attention paid to the concepts of reliability and validity.

As overall concepts, reliability is concerned with the consistency or repeatability of the results, tests or measurements used within research[1], while validity examines whether the research measures what it set out to measure and how applicable it is to a wider population[2]. Although sharing similar overarching principles in ensuring the accuracy and trustworthiness of research, reliability and validity are explored in different manners between quantitative and qualitative research.

RELIABILITY AND VALIDITY IN QUANTITATIVE RESEARCH

When applying the concept of reliability to quantitative research, we can consider reliable quantitative research to be that which utilises methods, instruments or measurements which will produce consistent results and the extent to which the results may be reproduced if repeated under the same conditions.[3,4] Assessing reliability allows us to appreciate how much variability in the measured results is due to errors in measurement, and how much is due to a true result.[5] Both reliability and validity are central elements to psychometrics and measurement.

High-quality quantitative research will demonstrate how the methods and measurement instruments chosen to answer the research question are reliable in obtaining consistent results. This may include selecting instruments that are previously validated as reliable or creating and then validating instruments with sufficient internal consistency, stability and equivalence, representing typical measures by which we may evaluate reliability. These are often examined using tests such as classic test theory or item response theory.

Internal consistency, or homogeneity, assesses how reliable a measurement is by estimating how well items within the measurement instrument are used to obtain the same results as other items assessing the same construct within the same instrument.[6,7] Stability examines the consistency of results using the same instrument, over time.[8] This can be assessed using methods such as test-retest and parallel-form reliability testing. Equivalence is concerned with the consistency among multiple users of an instrument, or the inter-rater reliability.[8] Equivalence allows us to understand how precise reported results may be and of what value they are in answering the research question.[8,9]

If we are satisfied that the results obtained are reliable, we must also consider whether they are valid. Broadly, the validity of quantitative research relates to how well the chosen methodology does, or does not, support discovering a true answer to the research question posed and whether the results can be extrapolated to our own setting.[10] We can subdivide validity in quantitative research into internal and external validity.

The internal validity of a study is concerned with how well a study controls extraneous variables to allow for the establishment of a causal relationship between the independent and dependent variable.[11] When evaluating the internal validity of a quantitative study, we must consider how appropriate the methodology is for answering the research question, whether the sampling and data analysis plans are appropriate and whether the stated conclusions match the reported results in the context of the sample obtained.[11,12] Threats to the internal validity of the study will inherently vary dependent on the research question and chosen methodology (see Table 18.1).

Although internal validity is a key priority in research, the importance of external validity in fields such as paramedicine cannot be understated.[13] External validity is concerned with whether we can apply results with good reliability and internal validity to patients within our own clinical setting.[14] To determine whether a study has sufficient external validity, we must consider whether the sample obtained in the research is generalisable to the population we serve in our current setting, paying particular attention to factors such as age, sex, presence or absence of co-morbidities and shared backgrounds.

RELIABILITY AND VALIDITY IN QUALITATIVE RESEARCH

The concepts of reliability and validity as they exist in the quantitative paradigm are perhaps unsuitable, or unwieldy, to apply to qualitative research.[15] While quantitative research follows structured and preset methods, in qualitative research, it is critical to remain flexible to developing themes in the research.[15] Despite this need for flexibility, it is important that we can be satisfied qualitative research is sufficiently rigorous, leading to the proposal by Guba and Lincoln of trustworthiness as a more applicable framework for assessing and preparing reliable and valid qualitative research.[16] Although there have been subsequent additional

TABLE 18.1 Threats to Internal Validity in Quantitative Research[11]

Threat	Rationale
History	Encompasses the events a study participant or researcher experiences during the research, including staff changes, symptom exacerbations or factors as simple as listening to news stories related to the research. Less likely to impact short-term research, but over longer term may impact study outcomes.
Maturation	Involves any biological changes occurring over time, including fatigue, wound healing and disease progression.
Testing	Testing may produce reactive responses from participants. Initial tests may provide clues to participants as to what the outcome of interest is, while during repeated testing, they may attempt to learn the 'correct' answers and modify their responses accordingly.
Instrument decay	The decay of any instrument used to measure outcomes is of concern to internal validity. Decay of an automated non-invasive blood pressure monitor in a long-term study of blood pressure control, for example.
Statistical regression	The concept of regression to the mean, in which participants who initially score highly on initial testing are likely to score lower the next time they are examined with or without intervention and vice versa. Thus, if participants are selected for research based on high or low scores, they will likely demonstrate a regression to the mean regardless of the intervention.
Selection	Potential bias in the selection of participants in the control and experimental groups.
Mortality	Includes not only mortality but study attrition and drop-out rate. May often be higher in experimental groups as these tend to require more commitment than control groups, leaving only highly motivated individuals in the experimental group and producing a skewed view of benefit.

Source: Flannelly KJ, Flannelly LT, Jankowski KR. Threats to the internal validity of experimental and quasi-experimental research in healthcare. Journal of Health Care Chaplaincy. 2018 July; 24(3):107–30. Online. Available: http://doi.org/10.1080/08854726.2017.142 1019.

criteria added to the original framework proposed by Guba and Lincoln, encompassing the domains of credibility, dependability, transferability and confirmability remains the most commonly applied.[16]

Credibility closely mirrors the quantitative concept of internal validity, as it relates to how the researcher demonstrates that the reported results are grounded in the reality of the participants' responses.[17] Taking steps to improve credibility in qualitative research ultimately ensures that the participants' voices are appropriately reflected in the research product (see Table 18.2).[17]

The concept of dependability is concerned with the repeatability of results.[21] However, the paradigm of qualitative research inherently lends itself to results that may not be reproducible.[21] Instead, dependability in qualitative research is focused on the stability and consistency of the methods by which the researcher has conceptualised the research, collected the data and interpreted the findings.[21]

Transferability in qualitative research shares similarities with external validity for quantitative research, in that it relates to the extent to which the study's findings could be applied elsewhere.[19] Ultimately, though, it is not the role of the researcher to demonstrate how their results can be applied elsewhere. Rather, it is their role to provide sufficient context and evidence to determine whether the results could be applied externally.[19]

Finally, confirmability seeks to establish how confident we are that the reported results are based on truth and not subject to the biases of the researchers.[20] Some argue that confirmability is demonstrated when credibility, dependability and transferability are sufficiently demonstrated.[20] In essence, when we consider whether the research demonstrates confirmability, we must ask whether another qualitative researcher working with the same data would draw similar conclusions.

EXAMPLE 1

Case Study

The air ambulance service you currently work with is considering implementing the use of thoracic ultrasound for the evaluation of pneumothorax during flight, as they have found that the use of a stethoscope is limited by the noise of the aircraft. They discover a study by Roline and colleagues which may assist in determining if this is a feasible option.[22]

In their study, Roline and colleagues performed a prospective feasibility study evaluating the use of point of care ultrasound (POCUS) during flight to evaluate lung sliding sign.[22] Although a useful tool, POCUS must be interpreted by clinicians and so suffers from variable inter-rater reliability. In their methods section, Roline and colleagues outline that clinicians in the study received a 15-minute

TABLE 18.2 Improving Trustworthiness of Qualitative Research

Guba and Lincoln Criteria	Strategies to Improve/Evaluate Criteria
Credibility[17]	• Accounting for personal biases before conducting research
	• Record keeping to demonstrate clear and transparent decision trail
	• Inclusion of verbatim participant accounts to represent perspectives
	• Respondent validation, or member checking, which involves inviting participants to comment on the themes identified and whether they feel accurately represented
	• Data triangulation, whereby the researcher may use multiple methods and data sources to gain a complete understanding of the phenomenon
Dependability[18]	• Performance of an inquiry/external audit, allowing an external researcher to review the data collection and data analysis and subsequently compare this against the stated results to confirm the accuracy of the findings
Transferability[19]	• Providing sufficiently detailed descriptions of the context in which the research was conducted to allow external researchers to consider applicability in their context
Confirmability[20]	• Establishment of an audit trail, recording details around unique topics during discussion and the rationale behind coding and thematic analysis
	• Establishment of reflexivity, an attitude that allows the researcher to understand how their background and position may influence the research process

Source: Noble H, Smith J. Issues of validity and reliability in qualitative research. Evidence-Based Nursing. 2015 April; 18(2): 34–5. Online. Available: http://doi.org/10.1136/eb-2015-102054.

lecture, participated in a 60-minute hands-on training session and demonstrated competency on a volunteer model prior to participating.[22] The use of standardised training is a recognised method for reducing the impact of equivalence on the reliability of quantitative research.

With these things considered, you decide that this study has sufficiently adjusted methods to reduce the impact of equivalence on the reported outcomes and continue to assess the validity of the study.

EXAMPLE 2

Case Study

You are reviewing the use of intravenous fluids in paramedic practice and considering the relative pros and cons of different formulations. You stumble across a study by Self and colleagues comparing the use of balanced crystalloids versus saline in non-critically ill adult patients in the emergency department.[23] You wonder whether this be applied to paramedic practice.

In their study, Self and colleagues conducted a single-centre, pragmatic, multiple-crossover trial comparing balanced crystalloids such as lactated Ringer's solution or Plasma-Lyte with saline among adults treated with intravenous crystalloids in the emergency department who were hospitalised outside the intensive care unit.[23] The primary outcome of interest was hospital-free days, with secondary outcomes including major adverse kidney events within 30 days, with a finding of no difference in hospital-free days (median 25 days, adjusted odds ratio 0.98, 95%CI 0.92–1.04, $p = 0.41$), and a lower rate of major adverse kidney events with the use of balanced crystalloids (adjusted odds ratio 0.82, 95%CI 0.70–0.95, $p = 0.01$).

On surface value, this study may have some relevance to paramedicine, as the patient population seen in the emergency department is not dissimilar to the population seen by paramedics. However, it is important when assessing for external validity to move beyond this general assumption. In their study, Self and colleagues examined a patient population with a median age of 54 (interquartile range [IQR] 37–67), equal sex distribution, a predominantly white background (78.2%), a moderate preexisting comorbid burden and generally suffering from medical complaints.[23]

Having examined the patient population studied within the research by Self and colleagues, you take this data away and compare it against the data available for your local service.[23] Finding that this population is similar to your current patient population, you consider that this study may have some external validity to your current setting.

CONCLUSION

It is paramount when conducting or critically appraising research that we are satisfied the results are consistent and precise, while ensuring the methods used to obtain these results logically assist in providing a true answer to the research question. Critical to achieving these goals are the concepts of reliability and validity. Although applied differently to accommodate the different paradigms of quantitative and qualitative research, reliability and validity are critical in ensuring the production and implementation of high-quality research.

REVIEW QUESTIONS

1. In your own words, define reliability and validity.
2. What are the variables to consider?
3. Describe the difference between internal and external validity.
4. Why are the concepts of reliability and validity evaluated differently in qualitative versus quantitative research?
5. What are the factors that impact internal validity?
6. What are the factors that impact external validity?
7. Discuss credibility and dependability in qualitative research.

REFERENCES

1. Al-Jundi A, Sakka S. Critical appraisal of clinical research. Journal of Clinical and Diagnostic Research. 2017 May; 11(5):JE01–5. Online. Available: http://doi.org/10.7860/JCDR/2017/26047.9942.
2. Patino CM, Ferreira JC. Internal and external validity: can you apply research study results to your patients? Journal Brasileiro de Pneumologia. 2018 May; 44(3):183. Online. Available: http://doi.org/10.1590/S1806-37562018000000164.
3. Matheson GJ. We need to talk about reliability: making better use of test-retest studies for study design and interpretation. PeerJ Publishing. 2019;7:e6918. Online. Available: http://doi.org/10.7717/peerj.6918.
4. Lachin JM. The role of measurement reliability in clinical trials. Clinical Trials. 2004;1(6):553–66. Online. Available: http://doi.org/10.1191/1740774504cn057oa.
5. Gosall N, Gosall G. The doctor's guide to critical appraisal. Cheshire, The United Kingdom: Pastest; 2015. p. 134.
6. McCrae RR, Kurtz JE, Yamagata S, Terracciano A. Internal consistency, retest reliability and their implications for personality scale validity. Personality and Social Psychology Review. 2011 Feb;15(1):28–50. Online. Available: http://doi.org/10.1177/1088868310366253.
7. Boateng GO, Neilands TB, Frongillo EA, Melgar-Quiñonez HR, Young SL. Best practices for developing and validating

scales for health, social and behavioural research: a primer. Frontiers in Public Health. 2018;6:149. Online. Available: http://doi.org/10.3389/fpubh.2018.00149.

8. Heale R, Twycross A. Validity and reliability in quantitative studies. Evidence-Based Nursing. 2015 July;18(3):66–7. Online. Available: http://doi.org/10.1136/eb-2015-102129.

9. Burns M. How to establish interrater reliability. Nursing. 2014 Oct;44(10):56–8. Online. Available: http://doi.org/10.1097/01.NURSE.0000453705.41413.c6.

10. Slack MK, Draugalis JR. Establishing the internal and external validity of experimental studies. American Journal of Health-System Pharmacy. 2001 Nov;58(22):2173–81.

11. Flannelly KJ, Flannelly LT, Jankowski KR. Threats to the internal validity of experimental and quasi-experimental research in healthcare. Journal of Health Care Chaplaincy. 2018 July;24(3):107–30. Online. Available: http://doi.org/10.1080/08854726.2017.1421019.

12. Leung L. Validity, reliability and generalizability in qualitative research. Journal of Family Medicine and Primary Care. 2015 Jul;4(3):324–7. Online. Available: http://doi.org/10.4103/2249-4863.161306.

13. Steckler A, McLeroy KR. The importance of external validity. American Journal of Public Health. 2008 Jan; 98(1):9–10. Online. Available: http://doi.org/10.2105/AJPH.2007.126847.

14. Murad M, Katabi A, Benkhadra R, Montori VM. External validity, generalisability, applicability and directness: a brief primer. BMJ Evidence-Based Medicine. 2018 Jan;23(1):17–19. Online. Available: http://doi.org/10.1136/ebmed-2017-110800.

15. Cypress BS. Rigor or reliability and validity in qualitative research: perspectives, strategies, reconceptualization and recommendations. Dimensions of Critical Care Nursing. 2017 Jul;36(4):253–63. Online. Available: http://doi.org/10.1097/DCC.0000000000000253.

16. Morse JM, Barrett M, Mayan M, Olson K, Spiers J. Verification strategies for establishing reliability and validity in qualitative research. International Journal of Qualitative Methods. 2002 Jun;1(2):13–22. Online. Available: http://doi.org/10.1177/160940690200100202.

17. Noble H, Smith J. Issues of validity and reliability in qualitative research. Evidence-Based Nursing. 2015 Apr;18(2):34–5. Online. Available: http://doi.org/10.1136/eb-2015-102054.

18. Forero R, Nahidi S, De Costa J, Mohsin M, Fitzgerald G, Gibson N, McCarthy S, Aboagye-Sarfo P. Application of four-dimension criteria to assess rigour of qualitative research in emergency medicine. BMC Health Services Research. 2018 Feb;18:120. Online. Available: http://doi.org/10.1186/s12913-018-2915-2.

19. Hadi MA, Closs SJ. Ensuring rigour and trustworthiness of qualitative research in clinical pharmacy. International Journal of Clinical Pharmacy. 2016 Jun;38(3):641–6. Online. Available: http://doi.org/10.1007/s11096-015-0237-6.

20. Korstjens I, Moser A. Practical guidance to qualitative research. Part 4: trustworthiness and publishing. European Journal of General Practice. 2018 Dec;24(1):120–4. Online. Available: http://doi.org/10.1080/13814788.2017.1375092.

21. Johnson JL, Adkins D, Chauvin S. A review of the quality indicators of rigor in qualitative research. American Journal of Pharmaceutical Education. 2020 Jan;84(1):7120. Online. Available: http://doi.org/10.5688/ajpe7120.

22. Roline CE, Heegaard WG, Moore JC, Joing SA, Hildebrandt DA, Biros MH, et al. Feasibility of bedside thoracic ultrasound in the helicopter emergency medical services setting. Air Medical Journal. 2013 May;32(3):153–7. Online. Available: http://doi.org/10.1016/j.amj.2012.10.013.

23. Self WH, Semler MW, Wanderer JP, Wang L, Byrne DW, Collins SP, et al. Balanced crystalloids versus saline in noncritically ill adults. New England Journal of Medicine. 2018;378:819–28. http://doi.org/10.1056/NEJMoa1711586.

19

Sampling

Kelly-Ann Bowles

LEARNING OUTCOMES

1. Describe the different sampling methods used in research

2. Identify the strengths and limitations of commonly used sampling methods

DEFINITIONS

- Population: Entire set of persons, objects or events in the research.
- Sample: The subgroup of the population included in the research.
- Sampling bias: The bias in the results when the sample does not represent the population.

INTRODUCTION

When it comes to finding an answer to a research question, it is not always possible to include every person from the entire population in the study. That said, most countries do hold some form of 'census' of their entire population on a scheduled timeframe, but these are very costly and time consuming. For example, the census in England and Wales is completed every 10 years with the 2021 census expected to cost £800 million and aiming for 94% of the population completing the form.[1] Australia currently completes a census every 5 years but with the great cost and resource requirements, governments are considering different methods to collect the data they need to help with population resource planning. This is a situation researchers are faced with every time they design a project. Much time is spent determining how to ensure we enrol a sample that is representative of the wider population, especially if we want to suggest that the results found in our research would be similar to that of the entire population (inference).

SAMPLING METHODS

There are two main types of sampling methods used when completing research. The first method is probability sampling (or random sampling) which is recognised by the fact that every person in the population should have a known and equal chance of being enrolled in the sample. It is the preferred method in quantitative research, especially if we want to infer the results of the sample to the wider population. The second method is non-probability sampling in which the researcher may select samples based on subjective judgments rather than a random selection. This method is often used in qualitative research or exploratory studies. Within each of these methods are a number of different strategies, with the main ones discussed next. For each strategy we will assume that the overall research questions is:

What is the effect of lower back pain in paramedics working in Australia?

Probability Sampling

- *Simple random sampling*: Basically, this is like pulling a number out of hat. To truly get a simple random sample I could use a random number generator, match the numbers to paramedic's registration numbers and then include these people in my sample.
- *Systematic random sampling*: Here I am going to apply a system to my sampling. Again I may use registration numbers but I may select every 100th number in order and include these people in my sample.

- *Stratified random sampling*: Factors like gender or age group may be related to lower back pain so I want to make sure that I have good representation from each group (strata) within these factors. First, I will divide all registration numbers into groups of factors that do not overlap but represent everyone in the population (e.g. females under 40 years of age, females 40 years of age or older, males under 40 years of age, males 40 years of age or older). I will then follow the process of simple random sampling to get numbers in each group that are proportionate to the population distribution (i.e. if 32% of all Australian paramedics are females under the age of 40 then I would prefer 32% of my sample to be in this group).
- *Cluster random sampling*: I decide that it is too hard to get to all paramedics so I decide to target ambulance stations. So instead of randomising the paramedic, I randomise the station (now known as a cluster). I will use simple or systematic random sampling to select my clusters and will then use one of those approaches again to sample from within the cluster.

Non-Probability Sampling

- *Convenience sampling*: As suggested, this involves including people in your research that are convenient. As I am designing my research, the professional body is holding their annual conference so I decide that I will get my sample by going to the conference and asking attendees to participate in my research.
- *Quota sampling*: Like stratified random sampling I acknowledge that there may be groups or strata important to lower back pain. So although the sample is still not random, within my convenience sample I am going to set quotas on how many people I want in each group of my sample.
- *Purposive sampling*: To do this well I need to know important information about my research. For example, I don't want to include any paramedic who has not had back pain so I purposely seek out those who have submitted a sick leave claim for lower back pain, and ask these paramedics to be in my sample.
- *Snowball sampling*: As the name suggests, in this strategy I include people in my study as they hear about it from

colleagues. So I send a survey to paramedics I know asking them to share it with their colleagues and it continues to get shared until I decide to close the study.

Although researchers may have a preference for one strategy over another, it is important to understand the objective of your research when you are considering your sampling method. It is very important that you understand your research question, to ensure that your sampling method allows you to answer the question in an efficient and effective manner while limiting bias as much as possible. Table 19.1 shows some key difference between the different strategies while giving examples of when each strategy might best be implemented.

EXAMPLE

In 2018 the British Medical Journal (BMJ) published a randomised controlled trial looking at parachute use to prevent death and major traumatic injury when jumping from aircraft.[2] In this trial participants were randomised into one of two groups: jumping with a parachute or jumping with an empty backpack. The results of the trial said that 'there was no significant difference in the rate of death or major traumatic injury between the treatment (parachute) and control arms (backpack)'.[2] However, the authors did note that there was a bias in their study as they were unable to include a sample from an aircraft that was moving or flying. The only aircraft that they did use was the one in Figure 19.1. So although their results were correct for their research, it would be unable to infer the results to those jumping from a moving or flying aircraft, as their sample did not represent the conditions of this wider aircraft population.

CONCLUSION

Sampling is one of the most important aspects of your research methodology. Poor sampling can lead to bias in your results and an inability to infer your findings to a wider population. There are a large number of sampling methods, and researchers should assess the advantages and disadvantages of each of these methods when designing their research project.

TABLE 19.1   Key Factors that Differ Between Probability and Non-Probability Sampling Methods

Type of Sampling	When to Use it	Advantages	Disadvantages
Probability Sampling			
Simple random sampling	When the population members are similar to one another on important variables	Ensures a high degree of representativeness	Time consuming and tedious
Systematic sampling	When the population members are similar to one another on important variables	Ensures a high degree of representativeness, and no need to use a table of random numbers	Less random than simple random sampling
Stratified random sampling	When the population is diverse and contains different groups, some of which are related to the topic	Ensures a high degree of representativeness of all the strata or layers in the population	Time consuming and tedious
Cluster sampling	When the population consists of units rather than individuals	Easy and convenient	Members of units may be different from one another, decreasing the effectiveness
Non-probability Sampling			
Convenience sampling	When the members of the population are convenient to sample	Convenient and inexpensive	Degree of generalisability is questionable
Quota sampling	When strata are present and stratified sampling is not possible	Ensures some degree of representativeness of all the strata in the population	Degree of generalisability is questionable
Purposive sampling	When there is a set group of people you wish to include in the study	Efficient, as you only include those relevant to your research	Requires strong knowledge of the research area
Snowball sampling	When the population is not known or information on the population is not readily available	Fast, cost-effective and good for populations that have hesitant persons	Sampling bias as recruitment may be limited to similar groups

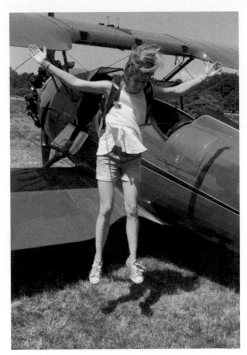

Figure 19.1 Aircraft that participants jumped from in the BMJ parachute trial. (Source: Yeh RW, Valsdottir LR, Yeh MW, Shen C, Kramer DB, Strom JB, et al. Parachute use to prevent death and major trauma when jumping from aircraft: randomized controlled trial. BMJ. 2018;363.)

REVIEW QUESTIONS

1. You are completing a study that is looking at the effect of an exercise program on cholesterol levels in paramedics. You have been told that a family history of high cholesterol levels could affect the results of your project. Which sampling strategy would be good to use in your project?

2. You are completing a qualitative project where you want to understand the lived experience of paramedics who have worked in remote communities. Which sampling strategy would be good to use in your project?

SUGGESTED FURTHER READING:

QuestionPro. Types of sampling: sampling methods with examples. Online. Available: https://www.questionpro.com/blog/types-of-sampling-for-social-research/.

REFERENCES

1. Barton C. Briefing paper: Preparing for the 2021 census (England and Wales). In: House of Commons Library, editor; 2021.
2. Yeh RW, Valsdottir LR, Yeh MW, Shen C, Kramer DB, Strom JB, et al. Parachute use to prevent death and major trauma when jumping from aircraft: randomized controlled trial. BMJ. 2018;363.

20

Power and Sample Size Calculations

Kelly-Ann Bowles

LEARNING OUTCOMES

1. Identify the difference between a null and alternate hypothesis
2. Identify the difference between type I and type II errors
3. Understand the importance of statistical power
4. Calculate a sample size for a simple research project

INTRODUCTION

As was discussed in the previous chapter, it is rarely possible to include an entire population in a research project. If it is possible to gain a census of the entire population, that is always preferable; however, feasibility constraints may make this very difficult. Therefore, in most quantitative research designs, the researcher aims to only include a sample of the population and then infer these results on the entire population. A very important question then focuses on how large this sample of the population would have to be. If your sample is too small, it may be biased and you may not be able to infer your results to the wider population accurately. If the sample size is too big, the research may be too costly or time-consuming, affecting feasibility. People have published entire books on the concept of sampling and power analysis, so this chapter will provide you with foundation information so that you can understand why it is important to determine the required sample sizes and the resultant 'power' within your research design in the early stages of your research.

HYPOTHESIS TESTING

In most quantitative research we should start with establishing a hypothesis. This is a clear, testable statement that the researcher expects to occur in their research. When we develop a hypothesis, we start with a null hypothesis. In single sample research (such as a survey of mean paramedic career length) our null hypothesis will be what the researcher expects to find (i.e. mean career length is 7 years). Our alternative hypothesis will then be the contrast of this finding (i.e. mean career length does not equal 7 years). In two-sample or comparative research, the null hypothesis should state that there is no difference between the two groups in your main outcome measure, and the alternate hypothesis would see a difference. This concept is important as errors can occur when we reject or fail to reject a null hypothesis (as can be seen in Figure 20.1) and sample size and statistical power can influence the likelihood of these errors occurring.

STATISTICAL POWER

The power of a research study refers to the ability to detect a difference if one does exist, or the probability of correctly rejecting a null hypothesis. As can be seen in Figure 20.1, a type II error occurs when we fail to reject a null hypothesis that is in effect false. The probability of a type II error occurring is referred to as beta (β) and the power is $1 - \beta$, as our research design is aiming to have enough power so that a type II error will not occur. The power of your research should be determined before you start as 'checking' your power retrospectively (also called post hoc power analysis) is flawed.[1] There are a number of factors that will affect the power of the research including: the effect size (how big a difference you are expecting between your groups; look in the Suggested further reading by Sullivan et al); the alpha (α) level (or significance level we are looking for, often 95%); and the sample size.[2]

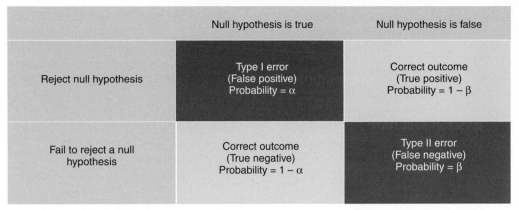

Figure 20.1 Type I and Type II errors when testing our hypothesis (modified from https://www.scribbr.com/statistics/type-i-and-type-ii-errors/)

SAMPLE SIZE CALCULATIONS

Sample size calculations differ depending on your research question and research design. If you are completing a cross-sectional study, like a survey, your approach to your sample size calculation will be very different than that of a randomised controlled trial. Regardless of your research design, the first step in determining the sample size is to establish the primary outcome measure of the research. It is very important to establish the unique primary outcome of your research as it is this measure that the sample size will be based on and from which you can set your hypothesis.

It is a good idea to review the literature in your area of research when starting to think about your sample size. Not only will this potentially give you some important information that can help you establish your own sample size, it is a good way to make sure that you do not repeat the same mistakes that others have made in the past.

There are different tables, websites and applications that can also help you calculate the sample size for a research study. These are found online or published in statistics textbooks. There are some criteria that you will need to know to work out your sample size. These criteria are then entered into established formulas that you can use to calculate your sample size. We will use a research example to calculate our required sample size using two simple formulas.

EXAMPLE

You are completing a research study to determine the prevalence (or proportion) of paramedics internationally who have suffered a back injury at work during their career. You start by determining your criteria.[3]

1. Confidence level: There will always be an amount of error or uncertainty in your results and we represent this sampling error with a confidence level. Often this confidence level is set at 90–95%, which means that if I repeat the research on different samples over and over again, I would be confident that in 90–95% of the trials I would get the same result.

2. Level of precision: This is effectively the precision you are willing to accept in your research. It is a range that the true value will be within. If we set a level of precision at 5%, and our outcome measure in our example says that 55% of paramedics have suffered a back injury, I am confident that the true proportion of paramedics that have suffered a back injury is between 50 and 60%.

3. Degree of variability: This is the distribution of the outcome we are measuring. From a conservative level we tend to set the degree of variability at 0.5 as this indicates the maximum variability in our outcomes. The more diverse our population, the greater variability we would expect. We then input these values into our formula.

1. *Cochran's formula*: This formula is best used on a large population. The formula is:

$$n_0 = \frac{Z^2 pq}{e^2}$$

Here:

n_0 is the sample size

Z is the number that you find in the Z tables of your statistics books and is related to the confidence level you select (95% confidence – $Z = 1.960$)

p is the degree of variability and q is $1 - p$. We are setting our variability at 0.5 so both p and q will be 0.5

e is the level of precision you select = 5% or 0.05;

$$n_0 = \frac{1.960^2(0.5)(0.5)}{(0.05)^2} = \frac{0.9604}{0.0025} = 384.16$$

so from this formula I would need 385 participants.

2. *Yamane's formula*: This formula is for smaller sample sizes so maybe the research is now being conducted in one area with 1000 paramedics:

$$n = \frac{N}{1 + N(e)^2}$$

Here:

n is the sample size

N is the population size for our research question (1000);

e is the level of precision you select = 5% or 0.05.

$$n = \frac{1000}{1 + 1000(0.05)^2} = \frac{1000}{3.5} = 285.7$$

so from this smaller population formula I would need 286 participants.

It is important to remember that formulas like those in this chapter do assume that we use simple random sampling (as discussed in Chapter 19) in our research and if you use other sampling techniques, like stratification, these calculations are a bit more complicated. Other sample size formula include criteria such as standard deviations (which you can base off others' research or your pilot testing), so it is good to understand the criteria you have available and the type of research you are completing when determining your sample size.

Once you have your sample size you should always factor in things like drop-outs or non-response. It is fairly common to increase your sample by approximately 10% to decrease the effect of drop-outs or non-response, but your review of the previous literature would be a good point to see if similar research had higher drop-out or non-response rates.

In qualitative research, sample size may not be as important because qualitative findings are not usually established to infer on a wider population. That said, it is important that qualitative researchers ensure diversity in the sample, relative to their research question. Traditionally it had been thought that qualitative researchers should seek to establish 'saturation' in their responses, meaning that no new ideas are given in subsequent interviews or focus groups. It is now felt that this concept may not be correct.

Ensuring that the sample is diverse and that the data answers the research question should give a qualitative researcher confidence that they have an appropriate sample.

CONCLUSION

To ensure that our research truly adds to the body of evidence, we need to be confident in our results. Having sufficient power and an appropriate sample size will give us confidence that we have decreased the probability of making an error in the interpretation of our results, and therefore our research can add to evidence-based decisions.

REVIEW QUESTIONS

1. If I fail to reject a false null hypothesis, what type of error would this be?
2. What factors affect the power of my research?
3. Is sample size important for all types of research?

SUGGESTED FURTHER READING

G*Power website: https://www.psychologie.hhu.de/arbeitsgruppen/allgemeine-psychologie-und-arbeitspsychologie/gpower.html.

Noordzij M, Tripepi G, Dekker FW, Zoccali C, Tanck MW, Jager KJ. Sample size calculations: basic principles and common pitfalls. Nephrology Dialysis Transplantation. 2010 May;25(5): 1388–93. Online. Available: https://doi.org/10.1093/ndt/gfp732

Sullivan GM., Feinn R. Using effect size—or why the *P* value is not enough. Journal of Graduate Medical Education. 2012;4(3):279-82. Online. Available: https://doi.org/10.4300/JGME-D-12-00156.1.

REFERENCES

1. Baguley T. Understanding statistical power in the context of applied research. Applied Ergonomics. 2004;35(2):73–80.
2. Rossi JS. Statistical power analysis. In: Schinka JA, Velicer WF, Weiner IB, editors. Handbook of psychology: research methods in psychology. John Wiley & Sons, Inc.; 2013. pp. 71–108.
3. Israel GD. Determining sample size. University of Florida Cooperative Extension Service, Institute of Food and Agriculture Sciences, EDIS, Florida; 1992.

21

Assessing Bias

Richard Armour and Brett Williams

LEARNING OUTCOMES

1. Define the concept of bias as it applies to research
2. Identify the tools that may be implemented to assess for the risk of bias in the published literature
3. Examine the common types of bias that may be present in both quantitative and qualitative research
4. Propose methods by which bias may be minimised in the conduct of research

INTRODUCTION

Bias refers to any systematic error, or deviation from the truth, in the results of inferences of a study.[1] The concept of bias must be denoted from the concept of imprecision, which is concerned with a random error rather than systematic error.[2] Biases may ultimately cause an underestimation or overestimation of the true effect of an intervention, although it is impossible to quantify the extent to which biases may have impacted the result.[1]

When conducting research, the methodology should sufficiently minimise the risk of common biases, and where it is not possible to eliminate a bias it should be explicitly acknowledged in the limitations section. However, when reviewing research, it is not acceptable to rely on authors to report possible sources of bias. Researchers should comprehensively review each manuscript to assess the methods by which authors have minimised the risk of bias in their research.

TOOLS TO ASSESS FOR RISK OF BIAS

To standardise the approach to assessing bias, several tools have been developed that provide frameworks for the assessment of the risk of bias across a number of study designs (see Table 21.1). Each tool is accompanied by a unique guide for its use to support effective implementation.

TABLE 21.1 Tools for Assessing Risk of Bias

Study Type	Recommended Tool(s)
Quantitative systematic reviews	• ROBIS[3] • AMSTAR 2[4] • COSMIN[5]
Randomised controlled trial	• RoB 2[6]
Non-randomised quantitative studies	• ROBINS-I[7] • Newcastle-Ottawa Scale[8]
Qualitative systematic reviews	• GRADE-CERQual[9]
Qualitative research	• CASP Qualitative Research Checklist[10,11] • JBI Critical Appraisal Checklist for Qualitative Research[10,11]

COMMON SOURCES OF BIAS

It is important to note that particular study designs do not inherently protect against bias. For instance, the randomisation process in a randomised controlled trial does not prevent all forms of bias, and so the research may still be rendered invalid by bias. The number of possible sources of bias is extensive, with some biases also having multiple names, and so here we will examine some of the more common biases in research.

Attrition Bias

Attrition bias is a subset of selection bias and may occur because of systematic differences between patients lost from the exposure and control groups through withdrawals, dropouts, loss to follow-up or protocol deviations.[12,13] To avoid attrition bias impacting research, researchers may elect to over-enrol in both treatment and control groups, or implement post-hoc strategies such as tailored replenishment samples and sampling weights.[13] When reviewing research, it is important to compare the demographics of patients lost from intervention and control groups.

Classification Bias

Also known as information or measurement bias, classification bias occurs when the accuracy of information collected is disparate between exposure and control groups.[14] This could refer to either misclassification of exposure or outcome data relevant to the research question.[14] Classification bias will produce an incorrect estimation of the association between an exposure and outcome.[15] Efforts should be made to reduce the risk of classification bias by using standardised measuring instruments, using multiple sources of information to classify groups, collecting data prospectively wherever possible and minimising the possibility of observation or recall bias.[15]

Confounding Bias

Confounding occurs when the effects of the exposure under study are mixed with the effects of an additional known or unknown factor, which ultimately distorts the true result.[15] Confounding bias may demonstrate an association where none exists or fail to establish a relationship where one does exist.[16] To mitigate the risk of confounding bias, it is important the researchers identify confounders that may impact the exposure under study, such as comorbidities, adjust for these confounders in analyses, or restrict confounders from being included, and report both crude and adjusted analyses to examine the impact of confounders on the true result.[16,17]

Friendliness Bias

Also known as acquiescence, directional or agreement bias, friendliness bias describes the tendency of participants to answer in the affirmative regardless of the actual question posed.[18] Common in research methods utilising survey instruments, friendliness bias may conversely manifest as a disaquiescence bias whereby the respondent exclusively responds in the negative.[19] This may ultimately result in an excessively positive or negative result or association.[19] If a researcher plans to use survey instruments in their project, it is important to avoid (wherever possible), questions with binary choices and ensure the questions selected do not imply a 'correct' or 'preferred' answer.[19]

Observation Bias

Observation bias is a result of a systematic difference between the true value and the value recorded by the observer.[20] This could range from different reporting of medical images, to different observers rounding up or down observations. Important measures to minimise observation bias include providing standardised training, making outcome adjudicators aware of their own preconceived biases and blinding outcome adjudicators to exposure status.[20,21]

Performance Bias

Performance bias may occur as a result of knowledge-of-intervention allocation by either the clinician or participant, with this knowledge resulting in disparate treatments between the intervention and control groups.[22] Performance bias may overestimate the benefit of an intervention by encouraging the participant or clinician to support the intervention with additional measures or to introduce additional interventions if the patient is in the control group.[22,23] Performance bias is mitigated by blinding at least the participants and clinicians to participant allocation as often as feasible.[23]

Publication Bias

Publication bias can have a significant impact on the overall state of paramedic literature and is particularly important to consider when performing systematic reviews, meta-analyses or writing clinical practice guidelines. Publication bias occurs from the selective publication of research based on the ultimate positive outcome of the study, rather than the quality of methodology.[24] This may potentially lead to a dearth of published negative trials, which when summarising the literature may paint an overly positive view of a given intervention. It is important for this reason that those seeking to summarise the literature examine more than journal article repositories. Instead, researchers should also include sources such as trial registries, conference proceedings and relevant regulatory documents.

Recall Bias

Recall bias most commonly occurs in case-control and retrospective cohort studies reliant on participants independently recalling their exposure status.[1] The ability of participants to accurately recall details is heavily influenced by subsequent events and outcomes.[1,25] The most effective way to avoid recall bias is to perform prospective research; however, when this is not possible, it is important that researchers carefully select research questions and avoid language that influences the participant answers.[25]

Selection Bias

Selection bias arises from any error in the selection of study participants and as a consequence of this error, the relationship between exposure and outcome differs compared against the wider, non-sampled population.[26] Ultimately, this means the results of the research cannot be applied to the wider population of interest. For this reason, it is important to compare the exposure and control groups' baseline characteristics for similarity and applicability to an external population, while also reporting on the methods of randomisation and blinding to interventions status.

EXAMPLES

Case 1

You are considering recommending a move from physician-authorised to autonomous paramedic fibrinolysis in the treatment of ST-elevation myocardial infarction (STEMI) and are reviewing the article by Davis and colleagues.[27] Davis and colleagues reported that the provision of fibrinolysis by autonomous paramedics was safe and feasible; however, you know that outcomes of patients suffering from STEMI may be impacted by a number of preexisting factors, and so are concerned about selection bias.[27]

In their study, Davis and colleagues examined pre-and post-intervention cohorts of patients with STEMI receiving prehospital fibrinolysis to compare the safety and feasibility of autonomous paramedic-delivered fibrinolysis.[27]

Because Davis and colleagues utilised a historical control cohort, this study had a high possibility of selection bias impacting the similarity between this historical control cohort and prospective interventional cohort.[27] However, Davis and colleagues were able to report and contrast key demographics and clinical features of the patients in both groups, finding no statistically significant differences.[27] This suggests that pre- and post-intervention groups were generally similar and unlikely to be subject to significant selection bias.

With this considered, you move on to consider the external validity of this research and additional methodological components of your critical appraisal.

Case 2

You are hoping to encourage active participation in research by paramedics in your local ambulance service. During your readings around this topic, you consider the article by Lazarus and colleagues examining the attitudes of paramedics towards enrolling patients in the PARAMEDIC2 trial.[28]

Following the completion of the PARAMEDIC2 trial examining adrenaline for patients with out-of-hospital cardiac arrest (OHCA), Lazarus and colleagues sought to examine the experience and attitudes of paramedics towards enrolling patients in research.[28]

Lazarus and colleagues distributed a questionnaire combining closed- and open-ended questions to paramedics involved with enrolling patients in PARAMEDIC2.[28] This questionnaire was distributed one month following the completion of enrolment for PARAMEDIC2; however, this was three years since enrolment commenced. As acknowledged by the authors, this placed responses at high risk of recall bias as it may have been a number of years since a paramedic last enrolled a patient in the research.

With this considered, you recognise the findings of the study as useful to understand attitudes of paramedics towards enrolling patients in clinical research, but acknowledge that there are likely additional opinions not encompassed by this research.

CONCLUSION

Bias may take many forms in research but is ultimately concerned with how significantly systematic, not random, error has impacted the reported results. Although it may not always be possible to eliminate all sources of bias when conducting research, it is essential these are identified and mitigated whenever possible to avoid over- or underestimation of the true intervention effect.

REVIEW QUESTIONS

1. Bias is a concern because:
   A. It makes the results of the research more difficult to read.
   B. It may ultimately cause an underestimation or overestimation of the true effect of an intervention.
   C. It may increase the precision of the results beyond what is needed.
   D. It may make the results imprecise.
2. When reviewing a randomised controlled trial, an appropriate tool to use to assess the risk of bias would be:
   A. ROBINS-I
   B. GRADE-CERQual
   C. AMSTAR 2
   D. RoB 2.
3. Describe publication bias and how it may influence evidence-based practice in paramedicine.

4. Confounding bias occurs when:
   A. research is selectively published based on the ultimate positive outcome of the study, rather than the quality of methodology
   B. participants answer in the affirmative regardless of the actual question posed
   C. participants are unable to accurately recall details about their exposure or symptom status
   D. the effects of the exposure under study are mixed with the effects of an additional known or unknown factor.

5. Publication bias occurs when:
   A. research is selectively published based on the ultimate positive outcome of the study, rather than the quality of methodology
   B. participants answer in the affirmative regardless of the actual question posed
   C. participants are unable to accurately recall details about their exposure or symptom status
   D. the effects of the exposure under study are mixed with the effects of an additional known or unknown factor.

6. Why is it important for investigators to take measures to reduce friendliness bias in their research?

7. Observation bias occurs when:
   A. there is a systematic difference between the true value and the value recorded by the observer
   B. participants answer in the affirmative regardless of the actual question posed
   C. participants are unable to accurately recall details about their exposure or symptom status
   D. the effects of the exposure under study are mixed with the effects of an additional known or unknown factor.

8. Performance bias occurs when:
   A. there is a systematic difference between the true value and the value recorded by the observer
   B. knowledge of allocation results in disparate treatments between the intervention and control groups
   C. participants are unable to accurately recall details about their exposure or symptom status
   D. the effects of the exposure under study are mixed with the effects of an additional known or unknown factor.

9. What implications would selection bias have on the results of a study?

10. Attrition bias occurs when:
    A. there is a systematic difference between the true value and the value recorded by the observer
    B. knowledge of allocation results in disparate treatments between the intervention and control groups
    C. there are systematic differences between patients lost from the exposure and control groups
    D. there is any error in the selection of study participants.

REFERENCES

1. Pannucci CJ, Wilkin EG. Identifying and avoiding bias in research. Plastic and Reconstructive Surgery. 2011 Aug;126(2):619–25. Online. Available: https://pubmed.ncbi.nlm.nih.gov/20679844/.

2. Castellini G, Bruschettini M, Gianola S, Gluud C, Moja L. Assessing imprecision in Cochrane systematic reviews: a comparison of GRADE and Trial Sequential Analysis. Systematic Reviews. 2018 Jul;7:110. Online. Available: http://doi.org/10.1186/s13643-018-0770-1.

3. Whiting P, Savović J, Higgins JP, Caldwell DM, Reeves BC, Shea B, et al. ROBIS: a new tool to assess risk of bias in systematic reviews was developed. Journal of Clinical Epidemiology. 2016 Jan;69:225–34. Online. Available: http://doi.org/10.1016/j.jclinepi.2015.06.005.

4. Shea BJ, Reeves BC, Wells G, Thuku M, Hamel C, Moran J, et al. AMSTAR 2: a critical appraisal tool for systematic reviews that include randomised or non-randomised studies of healthcare interventions, or both. BMJ. 2017 Sep;358:j4008. Online. Available: http://doi.org/10.1136/bmj.j4008.

5. Mokkink L, de Vet H, Prinsen C, Patrick C, Alonso D, Bouter L, et al. COSMIN Risk of Bias checklist for systematic reviews of patient-reported outcome measures. Quality of Life Research. 2018;27:1171–9.

6. Sterne JA, Savović J, Page MJ, Elbers RG, Blencowe NS, Boutron I, et al. RoB 2: a revised tool for assessing risk of bias in randomised trials. BMJ. 2019 Aug;366:l4898. Online. Available: https://www.bmj.com/content/366/bmj.l4898.

7. Sterne JA, Hernán MA, Reeves BC, Savović J, Berkman ND, Viswanathan M, et al. ROBINS-I: a tool for assessing risk of bias in non-randomised studies of interventions. BMJ. 2016 Oct;355:i4919. Online. Available: http://doi.org/10.1136/bmj.i4919.

8. Wells GA, Shea B, O'Connell D, Peterson J, Welch V, Losos M, Tugwell P. The Newcastle-Ottawa Scale (NOS) for assessing the quality of nonrandomised studies in meta-analyses. Ottawa: The Ottawa Hospital. Online. Available: http://www.ohri.ca/programs/clinical_epidemiology/oxford.asp.

9. Munthe-Kaas H. Bohren MA, Glenton C, Lewin S, Noyes J, Tunçalp Ö, et al. Applying GRADE-CERQual to quantitative evidence synthesis findings—paper 3: how to assess methodological limitations. Implementation Science. 2018 Jan;13(sup 1):9. Online. Available: http://doi.org/10.1186/s13012-017-0690-9.

10. Ma L, Wang Y, Yang Z, Huang D, Weng H, Zeng X. Methodological quality (risk of bias) assessment tools for primary and secondary medical studies: what are they and which is better? Military Medical Research. 2020 Feb;7(7). Online. Available: http://doi.org/10.1186/s40779-020-00238-8.

11. Majid U, Vanstone M. Appraising qualitative research for evidence syntheses: a compendium of quality appraisal tools. Qualitative Health Research. 2018 Nov;28(13):2115–31. Online. Available: http://doi.org/10.1177/1049732318785358.

12. Dumville JC, Torgerson DJ, Hewitt CE. Reporting attrition in randomised controlled trials. BMJ. 2006 Apr;332(7547):969–71. Online. Available: http://doi.org/10.1136/bmj.332.7547.969.

13. Nunan D, Aronson J, Bankhead C. Catalogue of bias: attrition bias. BMJ Evidence-Based Medicine. 2018 Feb;23(1):21–2. Online. Available: http://doi.org/10.1136/ebmed-2017-110883.

14. Lambert J. Statistics in brief: how to assess bias in clinical studies. Clinical Orthopaedics and Related Research. 2011 Jun;469(6):1794–6. Online. Available: http://doi.org/10.1007/s11999-010-1538-7.

15. Althubaiti A. Information bias in health research: definition, pitfalls and adjustment methods. Journal of Multidisciplinary Healthcare. 2016 May;9:211–17. Online. Available: http://doi.org/10.2147/JMDH.S104807.

16. Andrade C. Confounding. Indian Journal of Psychiatry. 2007 Apr;49(2):129–31. Online. Available: http://doi.org/10.4103/0019-5545.33263.

17. Haneuse S. Distinguishing selection bias and confounding bias in comparative effectiveness research. Medical Care. 2017 Apr;54(4):e23–9. Online. Available: http://doi.org/10.1097/MLR.0000000000000011.

18. Hinz A, Michalski D, Schwarz R, Herzberg PY. The acquiescence effect in responding to a questionnaire. Psycho-Social-Medicine. 2007 Jun;4:Doc07.

19. Kam, CC, Zhou M. Does acquiescence affect individual items consistently? Educational and Psychological Measurement. 2015 Oct;75(5):764–84. Online. Available: http://doi.org/10.1177/0013164414560817.

20. Mahtani K, Spencer EA, Brassey J, Heneghan C. Catalogue of bias: observer bias. BMJ Evidence-Based Medicine. 2018 Feb;23(1):23–4. Online. Available: http://doi.org/10.1136/ebmed-2017-110884.

21. Delgado-Rodríguez M, Llorca J. Bias. Journal of Epidemiology & Community Health. 2004 Jul;58;635–41. Online. Available: http://doi.org/10.1136/jech.2003.008466.

22. Mansournia MA, Higgins JP, Sterne JA, Hernán MA. Biases in randomized trials: a conversation between trialists and epidemiologists. Epidemiology. 2018 Jan;28(1):54–9. Online. Available: http://doi.org/10.1097/EDE.0000000000000564.

23. Spieth PM, Kubasch AS, Penzlin AI, Illigens BM, Barlinn K, Siepmann T. Randomized controlled trials—a matter of design. Neuropsychiatric Disease and Treatment. 2016 Jun;12:1341–9. Online. Available: http://doi.org/10.2147/NDT.S101938.

24. Dalton JE, Bolen SD, Mascha EJ. Publication bias: the elephant in the review. Anesthesia & Analgesia. 2016 Oct;123(4):812–13. Online. Available: http://doi.org/10.1213/ANE.0000000000001596.

25. Schmier JK, Halpern MT. Patient recall and recall bias of health state and health status. Expert Review of Pharmacoeconomics & Outcomes Research. 2004 Apr;4(2):159–63. Online. Available: http://doi.org/10.1586/14737167.4.2.159.

26. Tripepi G, Jager KJ, Dekker FW, Zoccali C. Selection bias and information bias in clinical research. Nephron Clinical Practice. 2010 Apr;115(2):94–99. Online. Available: http://doi.org/10.1159/000312871.

27. Davis P, Howie GJ, Dicker B, Garrett NK. Paramedic-delivered fibrinolysis in the treatment of ST-Elevation Myocardial Infarction: comparison of a physician-authorized versus autonomous paramedic approach. Prehospital Emergency Care. 2020 Nov;24(5):617–624. Online. Available: http://doi.org/10.1080/10903127.2019/1683661.

28. Lazarus J, Iyer R, Fothergill RT. Paramedic attitudes and experiences of enrolling patients into the PARAMEDIC-2 adrenaline trial: a qualitative survey within the London Ambulance Service. BMJ Open. 2019 Dec;9(11):e025588. Online. Available: http://doi.org/10.1136/bmjopen-2018-025588.

22

Culturally Inclusive Considerations in Paramedicine Research

Tom Davidson and Gemma Howlett

LEARNING OUTCOMES

1. Define key concepts within culturally inclusive research
2. Understand the key considerations when undertaking culturally inclusive research
3. Identify different strategies to ensure all research is culturally inclusive

INTRODUCTION

Multicultural societies such as the United Kingdom, the United States, Canada, New Zealand and Australia contain an increasing number of people from different cultural, religious, ethnic and linguistic backgrounds. It is crucial that researchers employ culturally inclusive approaches which take into consideration the issues and problems that are important for the people who are being 'researched'.[1] The aim of this chapter is to provide a brief overview of culturally inclusive research and to provide guidance to any researcher who wishes to undertake culturally inclusive research.

KEY CONCEPTS

Culture

When attempting to undertake culturally inclusive research, it is important to define the term 'culture'. Despite various uses of the term throughout the literature, culture generally refers to characteristics such as non-physical traits including values, beliefs, attitudes and customs that are shared by a group of people and passed from one generation to the next.[2] Research that is culturally non-inclusive will not consider the potential impact that culture can have on the research process or on the phenomena that is being researched.

In an increasingly globally mobile world, it will be rare to carry out research that does not have participants from different ethnicities, nationalities, political affiliations, socio-economic variances, sexual orientations, occupations and languages.[3] Groups cannot be thought of as a homogenous entity and all will have individualised understanding and experiences of a phenomena. It is therefore important to understand the collective impact of culture while appreciating the individual characteristics within the group. The key is to approach research in a way that is culturally inclusive for all. If research is targeted to a particular group, there still has to be an understanding of the diversity within this population.

Cultural Competence

Cultural competence based on cultural knowledge and cultural sensitivity is frequently emphasised in nursing research and practice. Cultural competence is the adaptation of a practitioner's approach in a manner that is consistent with the culture of the patient or service user.[4]

The Purnell Model for Cultural Competence helps healthcare providers understand potential components of culture (see Fig 22.1).[4] The model is a circle with an outlying rim representing global society, a second rim representing community, a third rim representing family, and an inner rim representing the person, the metaparadigm concepts. The interior of the concentric circles is divided into 12 pie-shaped wedges depicting cultural domains.

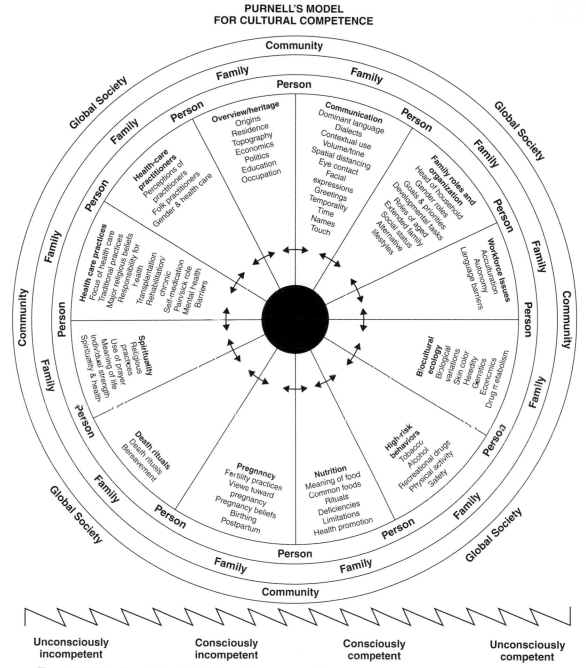

Figure 22.1 The Purnell Model for Cultural Competence. (Source: Purnell L. The Purnell Model for Cultural Competence. Journal of Transcultural Nursing. 2002;13(3):193–196.)

KEY CONSIDERATIONS

There is a significant amount of literature outlining the importance of culturally inclusive research, the pitfalls and how to do it properly. Table 22.1 provides an overview of some of the key considerations for researchers in cross-cultural research.

Culturally diverse patients are less likely to access healthcare in general due to various barriers including language, socioeconomic status, perception, understanding, distrust, confusion or fear. These same challenges will and can prevent participation in health research. Time and effort in relationship building with communities is essential when attempting to break down these barriers and include all people in any research.

Sensitivity is important in all stages, even if researching a defined group or culture. It is not possible nor necessary to make sweeping generalisable statements about those groups. Identity even within a similar population is often nuanced and complicated.[5] Identities such as immigration status, generational status, gender, socioeconomic status, sexual orientation, values and beliefs will intersect within a culture and lead to variance of experience and understanding of groups who may initially appear similar to each other.[5] An understanding of this and acknowledgment of variance in findings should be apparent in any research piece.

CONCLUSION

The paramedicine research profession is still relatively new, and it is vital that paramedicine researchers develop an ability to practice inclusively. This chapter has provided some examples of how to ensure inclusive practices within cross-cultural research. Just reading this chapter will not make readers inclusive practitioners and individuals needs to address all challenges and barriers to increase inclusivity in all areas of research and ensure that all communities and people are engaged with in a meaningful way.

REVIEW QUESTIONS

1. Think back on research you have planned or undertaken before. Was this research inclusive for all cultures?
2. Select a piece of research (this could be your own) and evaluate it against the sections within Table 22.1.
3. Use Purnell's model to explain the potential components of the cultures you may interact with.

TABLE 22.1	Key Considerations in Cross-Cultural Research
Consideration	**Description**
Previous experiences with research	Understand previous interactions with research/projects and how these were handled, understand any issues and ensure mistakes and bad practice do not happen again.
Interaction with community leaders	The creation of partnerships with community leaders and research participants is vitally important. Engagement and collaboration, if done well, builds trust and can help later in the process with any language barriers or translation.
Power balance	This includes inherent hierarchical structures and separation of those with education and those without. Every effort must be made to remove all power imbalance from the research process.
Research informed and shaped by the participant	Allowing leaders and participants to drive the research and help inform the research aims will demonstrate true engagement and collaboration.
Sensitive and appropriate	Educate all researchers on the communities, participants and cultural variances. Validate people's experience. Ensure accuracy, truth and sensitivity when portraying findings. Recognise the dangers of oversimplification of a group of people who will be joined by a culture but are all unique.
Barriers	Consider all barriers to participation, limit travel and carry out research collection in places people are familiar and comfortable with. Combat language barriers.
Action	Effort is required from the participants. It is important that they see action from research. Do something with the findings to make their investment worthwhile.

Source: Modified from Chakraborty J. Cross-cultural design considerations in healthcare. Lecture Notes in Computer Science (including subseries Lecture Notes in Artificial Intelligence and Lecture Notes in Bioinformatics). 2013;8005 LNCS(PART 2):13–19; Im EO, Page R, Lin LC, Tsai HM, Cheng CY. Rigor in cross-cultural nursing research. International Journal of Nursing Studies. 2004;41(8):891–9; and Delva J, Allen-Meares P, Momper S. Cross-cultural research. University Press Scholarship Online; 2010.

SUGGESTED FURTHER READING

Purnell L. Update: the Purnell theory and model for culturally competent health care. Journal of Transcultural Nursing. 2019;30(2):98105.

Im EO, Page R, Lin LC, Tsai HM, Cheng CY. Rigor in cross-cultural nursing research. International Journal of Nursing Studies. 2004;41(8):891–9.

Delva J, Allen-Meares P, Momper S. Cross-cultural research. University Press Scholarship Online; 2010.

REFERENCES

1. Cram F. Maintaining indigenous voices. In: The handbook of social research ethics (pp. 308-322). SAGE Publications, Inc.; 2009, pp. 308–322. Online. Available: https://dx.doi.org/10.4135/9781483348971.

2. Spector RE. Cultural diversity in health and illness. Journal of Transcultural Nursing. 2002;13(3):197–201.

3. Cleary LM. Cross-cultural research with integrity: collected wisdom from researchers in social settings. Palgrave Macmillan, Basingstoke; 2013.

4. Purnell L. The Purnell Model for Cultural Competence. Journal of Transcultural Nursing. 2002;13(3):193–196.

5. Delva J, Allen-Meares P, Momper S. Cross-cultural research. University Press Scholarship Online; 2010.

Explaining the What (Quantitative)

After you have considered why research is important and gained an understanding of the different frameworks and designs used (Section 1), and you have prepared for your own research (Section 2), it is time to consider quantitative research approaches. This section is called explaining the *what* and is distinct from explaining the *why*, which is discussed in the following section. The current section is divided into two different parts: the first looks at different quantitative research designs, followed by an introductory section to statistics and quantitative analysis.

Most people's research journey starts in the field after they have witnessed or reflected on something that is perceived as interesting or troublesome (and in need of repair) to them. Writing up these cases can be a great start and contributor to the literature (Chapter 23). Sourcing data from a larger subset of patients (or participants) but at a single time point can be useful and is the basis behind most survey studies (Chapter 24). Both case series and cross-sectional studies are limited by their inability to control against a baseline or someone without the disease, which is where case-control studies come to the rescue (Chapter 25). Further up the hierarchy of evidence, given the more robust data and decreasing chance of bias, is cohort and registry studies (Chapter 26). Although the gold standard of study types is the randomised controlled trial (RCT) (Chapter 27), it may not always be suitable for the research question at hand. In that case, some alternatives and modifications can be implemented (Chapter 28).

The data for your research project can come from many sources, hence consideration of their reliability and validity is important (Chapter 29). Being able to classify and visualise different data is important for analysing and presenting your findings (Chapter 30). Knowing how to handle missing data and the principles of hypothesis testing is important to consider before 'throwing' the data through the analyser (Chapter 31). Once you have established your null hypothesis, a *p*-value can be generated, but whether or not your results are statistically significant may or may not mean they are clinically significant (Chapter 32). When simple descriptive statistics and hypothesis testing is insufficient to answer the questions at hand, regression analysis (Chapter 33) and time-to-an-event analysis (i.e. survival analysis) (Chapter 34) may be used.

23

Case Reports and Case Series

Ben Meadley

LEARNING OUTCOMES

1. Define and differentiate between a case report and a case series investigation

2. Identify situations where a case report and/or a case series may be the most appropriate form of investigation

DEFINITIONS

- Case report: A detailed report describing demographic information, assessment, diagnosis, management and discourse of an individual patient.[1]
- Case series: A collection or series of case reports involving clinical situations where similar treatments or interventions were provided.[2]

INTRODUCTION

Healthcare professionals and research teams often encounter interesting clinical situations where some part of the patient care journey has generated a query or a line of further enquiry worth pursuing. Often, these situations may be reported in a case report or case series to share unusual or complex diagnoses and existing or novel interventions. These are often the beginnings of research projects that are on a larger scale and more involved.

Case studies and case reports are often how healthcare professionals are first exposed to research. An unanticipated clinical presentation, effect of an intervention or patient outcome may be seen as worthy of communicating and disseminating to the wider healthcare community. Further, a pattern in patient outcomes may evolve over a number of cases, revealing trends that may be significant for clinicians and researchers.

Table 23.1 summarises the major differences between a case report and case series. In a case report, there is the presentation of basic demographic information as well as the assessment, interventions and outcome(s). Other than descriptive information, there are not any statistical tests that can readily be applied, therefore limiting applicability to the wider population. For case series, detailed demographic information is described to ascertain the homogeneity or heterogeneity of the cohort. Further, detailed data

TABLE 23.1 Comparison of the Components of Case Report and Case Series Study Designs

	Case Report	Case Series
Number of patients	1	> 1
Basic demographic information	Yes	Yes
Detailed demographic information	No	Yes
Diagnostic information	Yes	Yes
Treatment	Yes	Yes
Outcome and follow-up	Yes	Yes
Statistical tests	No	Yes

regarding the assessments, treatments and outcomes are presented. Summarily, the major difference between a case report and case series is the ability to apply statistical methods to draw inferences from patient comparison.[3] In contrast to the case report, data may be generalisable to the wider patient community.

When considering writing a case report or a case series, protection of patient privacy is essential. Case reports are most often written retrospectively. Although approval from an ethics committee or institutional review board is not usually required, it is prudent to seek the advice of senior researchers in your health service (e.g. an ambulance service research department) before publication or presentation. Experienced researchers can guide the formulation of the case report and ensure that any content that may lead to patient identification is removed. More so, if there is an intention to detail information regarding the patient that may lead to identification and breach of privacy, then consent from the patient is required. In these instances, you must seek advice from your health service research department, and formal ethics committee or institutional review board approval may also be required.

As case series may occasionally be prospective studies, formal approval from both the healthcare research team and ethics committee or institutional review board should be sought at the outset. For the more common retrospective analyses, health service support and oversight should always be sought. As a rule of thumb, if more than three patients are to be included in a case series, then ethics committee/review board approval and support should also be sought.[4] If in doubt as to whether approvals will be required, be sure to ask the question before commencement.

EXAMPLES

Case Report

The research team presented a case of a 46-year-old male with a cough and fever during the COVID-19 pandemic. He had deteriorated over 5 days and his ambient air oxygen saturation was 56% with a respiratory rate of 46 breathsper minute and obvious dyspnoea. Despite 15 L/min of oxygen via a non-rebreather mask, the patient's oxygen saturation dropped below 90% on exertion. High-flow nasal oxygenation (HFNO) therapy was commenced, which was continued until admission in the intensive care unit. This case report discussed the feasibility of HFNO therapy in the out-of-hospital setting.[5]

Case Series

Preload and afterload reduction in patients with congestive heart failure (CHF) and acute pulmonary oedema (APO) is well established. Intravenous (IV) nitroglycerin demonstrates improved patient morbidity and mortality but is generally reserved for in-hospital management. In this study, the research team assessed the feasibility, safety and effectiveness of out-of-hospital IV bolus nitroglycerin in CHF with APO. The researchers reviewed all emergency medical services and hospital patient care records for CHF with APO and bolus-dose IV nitroglycerin. The median (interquartile range) systolic blood pressure was 211 mmHg (190–229), 5 minutes post IV nitroglycerin was 177 mmHg (155–199) and upon arrival at the emergency department was 181.5 mmHg (157–207). It was found that 94% of patients treated with IV nitroglycerin had CHF with APO. The case series found that patients who were treated by paramedics with IV nitroglycerin had improved systolic blood pressure and oxygen saturation upon ED arrival as compared to their initial presentation.[6]

STRENGTHS AND WEAKNESSES OF THIS DESIGN

Case Reports

Case reports are a good introduction to research for healthcare professionals. The inferences that can be drawn for the wider patient community from a single case are very limited; however, case reports are often an impetus and foundation for larger projects where results may be able to be generalised to the wider community.

Case Series

Case series provide more robust data for improvements in patient care. Patient demographics, treatments and outcomes can be analysed through established statistical methods, generating tangible results that may be generalisable to other patients. However, case series are retrospective studies that sit low on the hierarchy of evidence (see Chapter 13), and results should be interpreted in that context.

STEPS REQUIRED TO CONDUCT YOUR STUDY OF THIS DESIGN

1. Identify the clinical situation on which you may wish to report.
2. Seek advice and support from your healthcare service research team.
3. Determine if approval from an ethics committee/review board is required.
4. Use the guidelines provided by journals to formulate your study design (see Suggested further reading).

CONCLUSION

Case reports and case studies are useful research methods to form a foundation for larger research projects or to convey interesting or unusual patient clinical journeys. Although there are some methodological limitations, case reports and case series remain an accessible form of research for those not adept in complex biostatistical analyses and are an important part of the evolution of larger-scale research projects.

REVIEW QUESTIONS

1. What are the differences between a case report and case series?
2. Outline the required steps for writing and publishing a case report and case series.
3. Discuss when statistics in case reports and case series may be applicable and what the limitations of this are.

SUGGESTED FURTHER READING

BMJ Journals. For authors. BMJ Case Reports. 2021. Online. Available: https://casereports.bmj.com/pages/authors/.

Patterson PD, Weaver M, Clark S, Yealy DM. Case reports and case series in prehospital emergency care research. Emergency Medicine Journal. 2010;27(11):807–9.

REFERENCES

1. National Cancer Institute. Definition of case report. NCI Dictionary of Cancer Terms. National Cancer Institute. 2011. Online. Available: https://www.cancer.gov/publications/dictionaries/cancer-terms/def/case-report.
2. National Cancer Institute. Definition of case series. NCI Dictionary of Cancer Terms. National Cancer Institute; 2011. Online. Available: https://www.cancer.gov/publications/dictionaries/cancer-terms/def/case-series.
3. Ling S. Statistical methods for the analysis of case series data. Master of Science thesis: Dalhousie University; 2014.
4. Institutional Review Board. Case reports and case series. Boston University Medical Campus and Boston Medical Centre; 2021. Online. Available: https://www.bumc.bu.edu/irb/submission-requirements/special-submission-requirements/case-reports-and-case-series/.
5. Kedzierewicz R, Derkenne C, Fraudin A, Vanhaecke P, Jouffroy R, Jost D, et al. Logistical challenge with prehospital use of high-flow nasal oxygen therapy in COVID-19-induced respiratory distress: a case report. The Journal of Emergency Medicine. 2021 Jul;61(1):37–40.
6. Patrick C, Ward B, Anderson J, Rogers Keene K, Adams E, Cash RE, et al. Feasibility, effectiveness and safety of prehospital intravenous bolus dose nitroglycerin in patients with acute pulmonary edema. Prehospital Emergency Care. 2020;24(6):844–50.

24

Cross-Sectional Studies

Jennie Helmer

LEARNING OUTCOMES

1. Define cross-sectional studies
2. Understand the benefits and limitations of cross-sectional research
3. Recognise how cross-sectional studies can be applied to research in the out-of-hospital setting

DEFINITION

A cross-sectional study examines the relationship between disease (or other health-related state) and other variables of interest, as they exist in a defined population, at a single point in time or over a short period of time.[1]

INTRODUCTION

Cross-sectional study design is a type of observational study design where the investigator observes individuals without manipulation or intervention.[2] The participants in this type of study are selected based on particular variables of interest. Unlike other types of observational studies, cross-sectional studies do not follow individuals up over time. As well, unlike randomised control trials, which are experimental, the observational nature of cross-sectional studies permits the description characteristics that exist in a community, but not to determine the cause of something, such as a disease.[3]

Some of the key characteristics of a cross-sectional study include the following.

- The study takes place at a single point in time or over a short period.
- It allows researchers to look at multiple variables at once.
- The study can be used to look at the prevailing characteristics in a given population
- It can provide information about what is happening in a current population.
- It does not demonstrate cause and effect.

STRENGTHS AND LIMITATIONS OF CROSS-SECTIONAL STUDY DESIGN

Cross-sectional studies are popular in healthcare research but like other research designs they have strengths and limitations associated with their design and application.

Strengths of Cross-Sectional Study Designs

Inexpensive and Fast

Cross-sectional studies occur in a single point in time, compared to longitudinal studies, and are therefore usually inexpensive and easy to conduct, using self-reporting surveys and questionnaires. Another advantage relating to the speed of cross-sectional studies is that since data is collected all at once, it's less likely that participants will quit the study before data is fully collected.

Multiple Variables and Further Research

Researchers using the cross-sectional study design are able to collect data on multiple exposures and disease outcome simultaneously. This method of research also allows you to make correlations about possible relationships or to gather preliminary data to support further research and trials.

Limitations of Cross-Sectional Study Design

Do Not Demonstrate Cause and Effect

When using cross-sectional studies, you record the information that is present in the population of interest. Other variables can affect the relationship between the inferred cause and outcomes; therefore, cross-sectional studies don't allow for conclusions about causation.

Report Biases

Testing for associations and causality from cross-sectional studies must be interpreted with caution. Non-response is a particular problem affecting cross-sectional studies and can result in bias of the measures of outcome. This is a particular problem when the characteristics of non-responders differ from responders.

Cohort Differences

Groups studied can be affected by cohort differences that arise from the particular experiences of a unique group of people.

STEPS REQUIRED TO CONDUCT YOUR OWN CROSS-SECTIONAL STUDY[4]

1. Choose a representative sample.
   a. For generalisations from the findings to have validity, a cross-sectional study should be representative of the population. For example, a study of the prevalence of posttraumatic stress disorder (PTSD) among paramedics aged 30 to 40 years in a particular paramedic system should comprise a random sample of all paramedics aged 30 to 40 years in that system.
   b. The sample size should be sufficiently large enough to estimate the prevalence of the condition of interest.
2. Develop your survey. There are two types of cross-sectional surveys; descriptive and analytical.
   a. Descriptive cross-sectional surveys are purely descriptive and are used to assess the burden of a particular disease in a defined population. For example, a random sample of paramedics across a particular paramedic agency may be used to assess the prevalence of PTSD among paramedics who are 30 to 40 years old.
   b. Analytic cross-sectional surveys are used to investigate the association between a risk factor and health outcome. In this type of study, the risk factors and outcomes are measured simultaneously, and therefore may be difficult to determine whether the exposure proceeded or followed the disease status.
      In practice, cross-sectional studies will include an element of both types of survey design.
3. Conduct your cross-section study.
4. Analyse your cross-sectional study. The main outcome measure obtained from a cross-sectional study is prevalence.

a.
$$\text{prevalence} = \frac{\begin{array}{c}\text{number of cases}\\\text{in a defined population}\\\text{at one point in time}\end{array}}{\begin{array}{c}\text{number of persons}\\\text{in a defined population}\\\text{at the same point in time}\end{array}}$$

CONCLUSION

Cross-sectional studies are a useful research tool for out-of-hospital research. They can be considered as offering a snapshot of the frequency of disease or a health-related characteristic in a population at a given point in time. By learning more about what is going on in a specific population, researchers are better able to understand relationships that might exist between certain variables and develop further studies that explore these conditions in greater depth.

REVIEW QUESTIONS

1. Explain how the defining feature of a cross-sectional study is that it compares different population groups at a single point in time.
2. Compare and contrast the benefits of a cross-sectional study to other observational study designs.
3. Explain how cross-sectional studies cannot be used to determine cause and effect between exposure and outcome.

SUGGESTED FURTHER READING

Bigham BL, Jensen JL, Tavares W, Drennan IR, Saleem H, Dainty KN, Munro G. Paramedic Self-reported exposure to violence in the emergency medical services (EMS) workplace: a mixed-methods cross-sectional survey. Prehospital Emergency Care. 2014;18(4):489–94. Online. Available: http://doi.org/10.3109/10903127.2014.912703.

Power B, Bury G, Ryan J. Stakeholder opinion on the proposal to introduce 'treat and referral' into the Irish emergency medical service. BMC Emergency Medicine. 2019;19(1):81. Online. Available: http://doi.org/10.1186/s12873-019-0295-5.

REFERENCES

1. Rothman K, Greenland S, Lash T. Modern epidemiology. 3rd ed. Lippincott, Williams and Wilkins; 2012.
2. Hennekens CH, Buring JE, Mayrent SL. Epidemiology in medicine. Boston, Massachusetts: Little, Brown; 1987.
3. Black N. Why we need observational studies to evaluate the effectiveness of health care. BMJ, 1996;312(7040):1215–18. Online. Available: http://doi.org/10.1136/bmj.312.7040.1215.
4. STROBE. Strengthening the reporting of observational studies in epidemiology. 2022. Online. Available: https://www.strobe-statement.org/index.php?id=strobe-home.

25

Case-Control Studies

Alexander Olaussen

LEARNING OUTCOMES

1. Define and give examples of case-control studies within paramedic practice
2. Acknowledge and list the benefits and drawbacks of case-control studies
3. Recognise where case-control studies fit in the hierarchy of evidence
4. Be able to plan and conduct a case-control study

DEFINITION

A case-control study (or case-referent study) is an observational epidemiological study that compares a person (or group of people) that has an outcome of interest (e.g. a disease) with a cohort that is as similar as possible, but that does not have the outcome (i.e. the controls). While case-control studies traditionally have been labelled as retrospective, purely because the researcher is looking backwards having started by identifying the cases and then looking for potential risk factors or associated variables, oftentimes it is possible to do prospective case-control studies in which the identified cases and a suitable control cohort are followed forward.[1]

INTRODUCTION

A case-control study aims to look at variables that are potentially associated with an outcome of interest. The researcher first has to identify the cases (i.e. those with the outcome of interest) and then subsequently create a group of patients or individuals who do not have the outcome. This group will function as the controls or the reference group. Arguably the most significant case-control study in history was published in 1950 by Richard Doll and Bradford Hill on the association between smoking and lung cancer, in which they identified people with lung cancer and compared them to people without lung cancer.[2] Case-control studies sit low in the hierarchy of evidence due to its observational nature and risk of biases.

EXAMPLE OF A CASE-CONTROL STUDY IN PARAMEDICINE

Case-control studies can be suitable when studying rare disease or phenomena. For example, a senior paramedic wanted to learn more about a rare presentation: CPR-induced consciousness (CPRIC). He went to the Ambulance Victoria cardiac arrest database to try and find cases of CPRIC. Identifying the cases was the first challenge as 'CPRIC' was not a data field that existed. Therefore, searching through text words in the paramedic clinical notes was the start. Knowledge of a handful of cases enabled looking at those cases first to identify what kind of words would be used in this scenario by the attending paramedic crew. The search was reiterative, meaning that the search was repeated once a new potential keyword was identified. A list of several hundred potential cases was generated and those case reports were manually reviewed to try and identify whether the patient had regained consciousness during CPR (i.e. CPRIC), or whether these cases were falsely pulled from the registry because the words of interest related to either before or after the arrest (e.g. 'the patient lost consciousness and CPR was commenced' or 'the patient regained consciousness and CPR was stopped'). The final 112 cases were then compared to the 16,000 controls (i.e. the cases without CPRIC).[3] Figure 25.1 shows the abstract for this study.

Contents lists available at ScienceDirect

Resuscitation

journal homepage: www.elsevier.com/locate/resuscitation

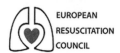

EUROPEAN
RESUSCITATION
COUNCIL

Clinical paper

Consciousness induced during cardiopulmonary resuscitation: An observational study☆

Alexander Olaussen [a,b,c], Ziad Nehme [a,d,e,f,*], Matthew Shepherd [a,f], Paul A. Jennings [a,b,f,g], Stephen Bernard [d,e], Biswadev Mitra [b,c,e], Karen Smith [a,d,e,h]

[a] Department of Community Emergency Health and Paramedic Practice, Monash University, Frankston, Victoria, Australia
[b] Emergency & Trauma Centre, The Alfred Hospital, Melbourne, Victoria, Australia
[c] National Trauma Research Institute, The Alfred Hospital, Melbourne, Victoria, Australia
[d] Department of Research and Evaluation, Ambulance Victoria, Doncaster, Victoria, Australia
[e] Department of Epidemiology and Preventive Medicine, Monash University, Melbourne, Victoria, Australia
[f] Department of Emergency Operations, Ambulance Victoria, Doncaster, Victoria, Australia
[g] College of Health and Biomedicine, Victoria University, Melbourne, Victoria, Australia
[h] Discipline of Emergency Medicine, School of Primary, Aboriginal and Rural Health Care, University of Western Australia, Crawley, Western Australia, Australia

A B S T R A C T

Background: Cardiopulmonary resuscitation-induced consciousness (CPRIC) is a phenomenon that has been described in only a handful of case reports. In this study, we aimed to describe CPRIC in out-of-hospital cardiac arrest (OHCA) patients and determine its association with survival outcomes.
Methods: Retrospective study of registry-based data from Victoria, Australia between January 2008 and December 2014. Adult OHCA patients treated by emergency medical services (EMS) were included. Multivariable logistic regression was used to determine the association between CPRIC and survival to hospital discharge.
Results: There were 112 (0.7%) cases of CPRIC among 16,558 EMS attempted resuscitations, increasing in frequency from 0.3% in 2008 to 0.9% in 2014 (p = 0.004). Levels of consciousness consisted of spontaneous eye opening (20.5%), jaw tone (20.5%), speech (29.5%) and/or body movement (87.5%). CPRIC was independently associated with an increased odds of survival to hospital discharge in unwitnessed/bystander witnessed events (OR 2.09, 95% CI: 1.14, 3.81; p = 0.02) but not in EMS witnessed events (OR 0.98, 95% CI: 0.49, 1.96; p = 0.96). Forty-two (37.5%) patients with CPRIC received treatment with one or more of midazolam (35.7%), opiates (5.4%) or muscle relaxants (3.6%). When stratified by use of these medications, CPRIC in unwitnessed/bystander witnessed patients was associated with improved odds of survival to hospital discharge if medications were not given (OR 3.92, 95% CI: 1.66, 9.28; p = 0.002), but did not influence survival if these medications were given (OR 0.97, 95% CI: 0.37, 2.57; p = 0.97).
Conclusion: Although CPRIC is uncommon, its occurrence is increasing and may be associated with improved outcomes. The appropriate management of CPRIC requires further evaluation.

Figure 25.1 Abstract for an example of a case-control study in paramedicine

STRENGTHS AND WEAKNESSES OF CASE-CONTROL STUDIES

The strengths of case-control studies lie in their ability to quickly and with a relatively low cost be able to investigate outcomes of interest. If a signal emerges from the data, this does not necessarily mean a causal relationship has been established, but rather that a hypothesis has been generated. Because case-control studies begin with identifying the cases, this study type lends itself well to investigating rare outcomes. Studying a collective group of patients with a rare outcome and examining potentially associated variables may provide the impetus for conducting further and more rigorous research into the potential for a causal link.

Another advantage of case-control studies is their ability to study multiple risk factors at one time.[4] A final advantage of case-control studies, and particularly relevant in 2020 regarding the COVID pandemic, is the ability of case-control studies to quickly study disease outbreaks.

One of the key weaknesses of case-control studies is that it is observational, meaning that any potential association is confounded by variables that are either unknown or known, but not measured. Another key issue with case-control studies is the veracity and reliability of the data in the exposure variables. As the data is often collected retrospectively and the subject may not remember, this introduces what is known as recall bias, or in some situations, the data registries may not be accurate or not have the data at all.

STEPS REQUIRED TO CONDUCT YOUR OWN CASE-CONTROL STUDY

Identifying the cases is the first step and the most important. While this might seem like an easy step, it may carry with it some challenges. Often the researcher wants to identify *all* the cases, which makes it difficult to be inclusive and specific at the same time. When studying CPRIC in the example just provided, the researchers could have chosen to only examine the dozen cases that they knew of personally. However, it was desired to study as many cases as possible to increase the power and statistical significance, to provide a stronger conclusion and to also explore trends over time—so a more rigorous method for identifying these cases was required.

The second step is to identify the control group. Depending on time and resources, this can be done in one of two ways. One could either grab all patients that are defined as non-cases or one could grab a matched sample, typically by a factor of two or more of the number of cases. For instance, the study on CPRIC identified 112 cases and then compared it to more than 16,000 other cardiac arrests that were not identified as CPRIC. Alternatively, those 112 cases could have been compared to a selection of patients that were similar in terms of age, downtime, initial rhythm and other important cardiac arrest outcome predictors. The former method is more robust but has the downside of being more labour-intensive and costly.

CONCLUSION

Case-control studies are a vital part of any speciality's body of literature. They should be conducted and interpreted for what they are, namely hypothesis generators and ways of looking for potential associations. Compared to other more rigorous study methods, they are quick and easy to perform; however, they rarely provide strong evidence for a causal link. They are observational and most often retrospective in nature, which demonstrates their major drawbacks in terms of the reliability and availability of the data obtainable.

REVIEW QUESTIONS

1. In 1950 when Doll and Hill published their report on smoking and carcinoma of the lung, a case-control study showing that there was a potential association between smoking and lung cancer met a lot of opposition. This resistance was based on the fact that this type of study could not provide evidence for causal effect. What out-of-hospital intervention are we doing today that the future will look at the same way, as we look at smoking and lung cancer today?

2. Identify three situations or scenarios (clinical or non-clinical) that would lend itself well to a case-control study. Consider the characteristics in which such a study methodology is suitable (e.g. rarity, data availability, cost, hypothesis-generating).

3. Where in the PICO/PECO format (see Chapter 6), would you place your cases of interest (e.g. CPRIC cases), when trying to generate a hypothesis? Hint: Not in P, as that would not allow for comparison.

SUGGESTED FURTHER READING

Armenian, H. The case-control method, vol. 38. Oxford University Press; 2009. Online. Available: https://doi.org/10.1093/acprof:oso/9780195187113.001.0001.

Equator Network (Enhancing the QUAlity and Transparency Of health Research): https://www.equator network.org/.

REFERENCES

1. Porta M, Greenland S, Burón A, editors. International Epidemiological Association sponsoring body. A dictionary of epidemiology. 6th ed. Oxford, England: Oxford University Press; 2014, p. 377.

2. Doll R, Hill AB. Smoking and carcinoma of the lung; preliminary report. British Medical Journal. 1950 Sep 30;2(4682): 739–48.

3. Olaussen A, Nehme Z, Shepherd M, Jennings PA, Bernard S, Mitra B, et al. Consciousness induced during cardiopulmonary resuscitation: an observational study. Resuscitation. 2017;113:44–50.

4. Tenny S, Kerndt CC, Hoffman MR. Case control studies. In: StatPearls. Treasure Island (FL): StatPearls Publishing; 2020. Online. Available: http://www.ncbi.nlm.nih.gov/books/NBK448143/.

26

Cohort Studies and Registry Studies

Hideharu Tanaka, Ryo Sagisaka, Koshi Nakagawa and Shota Tanaka

LEARNING OUTCOMES

1. Define cohort and registry studies
2. Recognise the characteristics of cohort and registry studies
3. Recognise the adaptation for cohort and registry studies in prehospital settings

DEFINITION

Cohort studies are a type of observational study design and registry studies is a generic term for database studies.[1] Cohort studies are studies that analyse 'a group of individuals selected for a particular purpose and tracked over a certain period of time' (e.g. exposed versus unexposed).[2] Registry studies are designed to deal with databases collecting patients' status and factors for specific purposes.[1]

INTRODUCTION

Cohort studies are classified as prospective or retrospective depending on the timeline of the study, while registry studies are generally retrospective.[2]

In prospective cohort studies, outcomes and predictors are observed from the present to the future for a fixed period of time from the initiation of the observation. At the same time as clarifying the incidence of outcomes, the temporal relationship between predictors and outcomes is evaluated. In addition, the strength of the causal relationship between multiple predictors and outcomes can be estimated. The measurement items are decided based on the study hypothesis before the start of observation.

In retrospective cohort studies, study objects are observed along a timeline, but databases that have already completed measurement on outcomes and predictors are analysed. The causal relationship between predictors and outcomes can be estimated. Measurements that are consistent with the hypothesis of the study may not be recorded.

In observational studies, real-world data are analysed, simple comparisons such as exposed versus unexposed cannot be conducted (i.e. the t-test or the chi-square test cannot be used to estimate efficacy). This is because confounders can distort the results and mislead them. There is a limit to causal inference because it can be affected by unmeasured factors.[3,4]

DIFFERENCES FROM CASE-CONTROL AND CROSS-SECTIONAL STUDIES

The difference from the case-control or cross-sectional studies in the previous chapter is the timeline of measurement.[2]

The case-control study is a retrospective study based on existing data. In studies targeting rare diseases, cohort studies are too time-consuming, expensive and inefficient. In such a case, case control is more appropriate, which evaluates the relationship between disease and predictors retrospectively.

The cross-sectional study measures at only one point. Unlike cohort studies, there is no follow-up period, so the merit is that the study ends in a short term. Since the purpose is to examine the prevalence (abundance rate) at the time of measurement, it is not useful for estimating causal inference.

DIFFERENCES BETWEEN PROSPECTIVE AND RETROSPECTIVE

Prospective

Because measurement items can be set prior to the start of the study, incidence and predictors can be measured, and temporal relationships are clear. Because a large number of subjects must be observed over the long period, they may drop out during observation, which can be costly.[2]

Retrospective

Because outcomes and predictors have already been measured, time and cost may be less than in the prospective cohort study. Since all measurements have been completed, it is impossible to control the method and content of measurements, and data can be incomplete or inaccurate.[2]

STEPS REQUIRED TO CONDUCT YOUR OWN STUDY OF THIS DESIGN

This time, you will consider a cohort study on adrenaline administration and survival for out-of-hospital cardiac arrest (OHCA) in the prehospital setting. Assume that you are already clear about which registry data to use. In this study, you will use the Utstein-style database, which is widely used in the world.

First, you will materialise the study using the PECO framework. In this case, you will use the following criteria—P: OHCA aged 18 years and older; E: adrenaline administration; C: adrenaline non-administration; and O: survival at 1 month. In other words, the purpose of the study is: 'Is adrenaline for OHCA in adults aged 18 years and older associated with survival at 1 month compared with no adrenaline?'.

Then you will extract the data that matches the purpose of the study. In this case, data inclusion and exclusion conditions are determined in advance. In this study, the inclusion criteria are all OHCAs aged 18 years or older, the exclusion criteria are outliers in the time sequence data (negative value) or incomplete data on treatment.

You will confirm the characteristics of the patient's data. Data are divided into adrenaline and non-adrenaline cohorts, and collected about information such as the age and sex of the patients. Next, you will analyse. As mentioned previously, the cohort study is influenced by confounders, so multivariable logistic regression analysis is used to estimate the relationship between adrenaline administration and survival at 1 month by adjusting for confounders. Factors that have been shown to have a relationship to outcomes in previous studies or that are clinically meaningful are selected and modelled. Be careful when you run the analysis. If you do not use the statistical model correctly, the results will be misinterpreted.

When writing a paper, you will typically present data extraction, patient characteristics data and the results of the univariable and the multivariable analysis. It is important to show all the results, not just the good ones, because it will mislead the reader. Observational studies are generally reported in line with 'STROBE' or ' RECORD'.[5,6] These were developed as checklists of items to be reported to improve the reporting quality of observational studies. It is also useful for reviewers, editors and readers to critically examine and interpret papers.

STRENGTHS AND WEAKNESSES OF THIS DESIGN

Strengths

It is possible to compare between those who received adrenaline administration in the real world and those who did not receive it. In general, the power is high due to using the large database. The results that can be widely generalised are obtained.

Weaknesses

Effects of unmeasured confounders may remain. Interpretation of results or conduction of analysis may be difficult if complex analysis methods are needed.

CONCLUSION

The cohort and registry studies are powerful study designs for assessing the social effects of exposures of interest using real-world data. On the other hand, if the data collection is retrospective, it is not optimised for research purposes and confounders may remain. In addition, multivariable analysis to correct for confounders is essential. Although it is not listed here, you should also use statistical models that suit your study purposes to address confounders. When these problems are cleared away, cohort studies and registry studies may provide a reasonable level of evidence.

REVIEW QUESTIONS

1. Define cohort studies and compare and contrast prospective and retrospective designs.
2. Outline the steps required to undertake your own cohort study and consider how you may overcome some of the challenges faced.
3. List a few reporting tools and discuss the benefits of adhering to these for the author, the reviewers and the editors.

REFERENCES

1. Mathes T, Pieper D. Study design classification of registry-based studies in systematic reviews. Journal of Clinical Epidemiology. 2018;93:84–7.

2. Rothman KJ, Lash TL, Greenland S. Modern epidemiology, 3rd ed. Lippincott Williams and Wilkins; 2012.

3. Howards PP. An overview of confounding. Part 2: how to identify it and special situations. Acta Obstetricia et Gynecologica Scandinavica. 2018;97(4):400–6.

4. Hartling L, Bond K, Santaguida PL, Viswanathan M, Dryden DM. Testing a tool for the classification of study designs in systematic reviews of interventions and exposures showed moderate reliability and low accuracy. Journal of Clinical Epidemiology. 2011;64(8):861–71.

5. Vandenbroucke JP, von Elm E, Altman DG, Gøtzsche PC, Mulrow CD, Pocock SJ, et al. Strengthening the Reporting of Observational Studies in Epidemiology (STROBE): explanation and elaboration. PLoS Medicine; 2007;4(10): e297.

6. Benchimol EI, Smeeth L, Guttmann A, Harron K, Moher D, Petersen I, et al. The Reporting of studies Conducted using Observational Routinely-collected health Data (RECORD) statement. PLoS Medicine; 2015;12(10):e1001885.

27

Randomised Controlled Trials

Ziad Nehme and Karen Smith

LEARNING OUTCOMES

1. Understand the strengths and weaknesses of randomised controlled trials
2. Recognise the four phases of randomised controlled trials
3. Identify the major components of randomised controlled trial design

DEFINITION

A randomised controlled trial is a prospective, comparative, interventional experiment where participants are randomly assigned to one or more interventions performed under controlled study conditions.

INTRODUCTION

Randomised controlled trials (RCTs) are the most rigorous scientific experiments for determining whether a causal relationship exists between an intervention and an outcome. The strength of the RCT is its ability to control for bias, which is the major pitfall of observational research. Bias is the deviation of results from the truth, which can be due to methodological issues involving the design, conduct, analysis or evaluation of results.[1] Data from rigorously conducted RCTs are the highest-level evidence for guiding decisions in the clinical environment.[1,2] However, a poorly conducted and biased RCT can lead to the adoption of clinical interventions that are costly, inefficient and potentially harmful to patients.

BIAS AND CONFOUNDING

In observational studies, there are often systematic differences in the groups being compared that give rise to false or misleading results.[1] *Bias* is a term used to denote systematic error in research methodology, which can occur when the selection of participants differs systematically or when the information collected differs across groups. Systematic differences can be the result of *confounding*, which is when a known or unknown risk factor is associated with both the intervention and the outcome. The gold standard approach for eliminating these systematic differences is to randomly allocate each participant into groups. In doing so, the probability of being allocated to a treatment group is determined solely by chance.

CONDUCTING CLINICAL TRIALS

Biased findings from poorly conducted RCTs can lead to the adoption of wasteful interventions and can have devastating impacts on health outcomes.[3] Conversely, a lack of confidence in the methodological quality of RCTs can delay the uptake of clinically important findings. There is strong evidence that the quality of reporting of clinical trials is not optimal, with incomplete and inaccurate reporting of trial methods present in as many as 80% of RCTs.[4] There is international guidance on the planning and conduct of RCTs, known as the CONSORT statement (Consolidated Standards of Reporting Trials). The CONSORT statement is an evidence-based minimum set of recommendations for reporting the design, analysis and interpretation of RCTs which is widely endorsed by medical journals.[2]

PHASES OF A CLINICAL TRIAL

Clinical trials evaluating the safety and efficacy of medications are typically tested in four sequential phases.[5] Phase 1 trials aim to determine the safety and side-effect profile of the intervention in a small, healthy human population. Phase 2 trials aim to determine the safety and efficacy of the intervention in a larger human population with the condition of interest (e.g. usually 100 to 500 people). Phase 3 trials are definitive studies of efficacy comparing the intervention with one or more other treatments in a large group of patients with the condition of interest (e.g. usually several thousand). Phase 4 studies are used to monitor adverse effects of an intervention in the post-marketing phase (e.g. general population use).

CLINICAL TRIAL DESIGN

The simplest and most common way to achieve randomisation in a clinical trial is the parallel-group design, where each participant is randomly allocated to only one of the intervention or control groups. By comparison, a crossover design will expose participants to both the intervention and control groups in a randomly allocated sequential manner. In doing so, the individual acts as their own control, eliminating the variation in group characteristics that might occur in the parallel-group design.[6] A more complicated design, called factorial designs, allows researchers to test the impact of two or more interventions in isolation and in combination when compared to a control. For instance, a 2×2 factorial design will randomly assign a participant to one of four groups: 1. a control group that receives no intervention; 2. an intervention group that receives treatment A; 3. an intervention group that receives treatment B; and 4. an intervention group that receives both treatments A and B. The factorial design is useful when researchers believe that the effect of one treatment may be influenced by another (i.e. an interaction) or where there is a desire to address multiple clinical dilemmas in the population of interest.[7]

RANDOM ALLOCATION

The random allocation of participants to one or more treatment groups is the cornerstone feature of an RCT. The role of randomisation is to achieve an equal distribution of confounding variables between the intervention and control groups. These confounding variables include key population characteristics (e.g. age, sex, preexisting conditions) and other prognostic factors which are known to influence the outcome. The most common approach to random allocation is called simple randomisation, which is analogous to a coin toss and is typically computer-generated.[8] 'Blocked' and 'strata' randomisation techniques can be used to ensure a balance of participants and their characteristics in each group, which is useful in smaller

trials. Cluster randomisation can also be used when individual randomisation is not feasible or practical.[9] In these circumstances, ambulance teams or hospitals can act as units of randomisation, where each unit is randomly assigned to either intervention or control. Random allocation is usually undertaken in a 1:1 fashion, meaning equal numbers of participants are randomised to the intervention and control groups. However, an unequal randomisation ratio may also be desirable, particularly if the cost of the intervention is high.[10]

ALLOCATION CONCEALMENT

One of the most common methods of concealing the participant's allocation to the treatment group is using concealed envelopes. This approach is common in the out-of-hospital environment and ensures that clinicians and participants are blinded to treatment assignment. Prior knowledge of a patient's treatment allocation can lead to bias by influencing the clinician's decision to enrol a patient in the trial.

BLINDING

Blinding is a methodological strategy used to reduce the risk of bias. Blinding is usually targeted at patients and their treating clinicians but can also include study investigators and statisticians. An open-label trial is one where both patients and their treating clinicians are aware of the intervention being provided. Single-blind and double-blind trials describe trials where either one or both parties (i.e. patients and their treating clinicians) are blinded to the intervention, respectively.

EXPLANATORY VERSUS PRAGMATIC TRIALS

While RCTs are the gold standard in research design, there are concerns that many RCTs do not adequately inform practice because they lack real-world generalisability.[11] Traditional RCTs, often termed 'explanatory trials', are designed to confirm a clinical hypothesis usually under very strict or controlled study conditions. Often the study population recruited can be highly selected and lacking generalisability, or the timing and dose of interventions may not reflect real-world practice. As a result, there is growing interest in the role of pragmatic trials in clinical research. Pragmatic trials are designed to inform clinical decisions by providing evidence of the effectiveness of the intervention under real-world conditions. The level of pragmatism in a trial is determined by the recruitment of investigators and participants, the intervention and its delivery, the nature of follow-up, and the nature, determination and analysis of outcomes.[12]

EXAMPLES

Prehospital Transdermal Glyceryl Trinitrate in Patients with Presumed Stroke (The RIGHT-2 Trial)

The RIGHT-2 trial was a multicentre, ambulance-based, randomised, phase 3 trial of glyceryl trinitrate (GTN) for the treatment of hypertension in acute stroke patients.[13] Patients were eligible for enrolment if they presented to paramedics with acute stroke symptoms within 4 hours of symptom onset. Patients were randomly assigned by paramedics to receive either transdermal GTN or a similar sham dressing in a 1:1 fashion using concealed treatment packs. Paramedics were unblinded to treatment, although patients were blinded since both dressings were similar in appearance. The primary outcome was functional outcome at 90 days after randomisation, measured using the seven-level modified Rankin Scale.

Mechanical Versus Manual Chest Compression for out-of-Hospital Cardiac Arrest (The PARAMEDIC Trial)

The PARAMEDIC trial was a pragmatic, cluster randomised open-label trial of mechanical versus manual chest compressions in the treatment of out-of-hospital cardiac arrest (OHCA).[14] Adults with non-traumatic OHCA were randomised by four United Kingdom Ambulance Services. Randomisation was conducted according to the first ambulance team on scene (clusters), which were randomly assigned (1:2) to either the LUCAS-2 mechanical device or manual chest compressions. It was not possible to blind paramedics to treatment; however, ambulance dispatch staff and those collecting the primary outcome were masked to treatment allocation. The primary outcome was survival at 30 days following cardiac arrest.

CONCLUSION

An RCT is the most scientifically rigorous method for establishing a cause-and-effect relationship between an intervention and an outcome. Although RCTs are useful for guiding decisions in the clinical setting, a poorly conducted RCT can lead to the adoption of clinical interventions that are inefficient and potentially harmful. International standards for reporting and conducting RCTs are now widely available and should be used by clinicians to interpret the quality of RCT evidence in the prehospital setting.

REVIEW QUESTIONS

1. What strengths do RCTs have over observational research?

2. True or false? All RCTs involve the randomisation of participants to only one of the intervention or control groups.
3. What are the four phases of clinical trials involving medications?
4. How does a cluster RCT differ from traditional units of randomisation?
5. True or false? A double-blind trial is when both patients and their treating clinicians are blinded to treatment assignment.

SUGGESTED FURTHER READING

Moher D, Hopewell S, Schulz KF, Montori V, Gøtzsche PC, Devereaux PJ, et al. CONSORT 2010 Explanation and elaboration: updated guidelines for reporting parallel group randomised trials. BMJ. 2010;340:c869.

Umscheid CA, Margolis DJ, Grossman CE. Key concepts of clinical trials: a narrative review. Postgraduate Medicine. 2011;123: 194–204.

REFERENCES

1. Kendall JM. Designing a research project: randomised controlled trials and their principles. Emergency Medicine Journal. 2003;20:164–8.
2. Schulz KF, Altman DG, Moher D. CONSORT 2010 statement: updated guidelines for reporting parallel group randomised trials. BMJ. 2010;340:c332.
3. Moher D, Pham B, Jones A, Cook DJ, Jadad AR, Moher M, et al. Does quality of reports of randomised trials affect estimates of intervention efficacy reported in meta-analyses? Lancet. 1998;352:609–13.
4. Hopewell S, Dutton S, Yu L-M, Chan A-W, Altman DG. The quality of reports of randomised trials in 2000 and 2006: comparative study of articles indexed in PubMed. BMJ. 2010;340:c723.
5. Umscheid CA, Margolis DJ, Grossman CE. Key concepts of clinical trials: a narrative review. Postgraduate Medicine. 2011;123:194–204.
6. Dwan K, Li T, Altman DG, Elbourne D. CONSORT 2010 statement: extension to randomised crossover trials. BMJ. 2019;366:l4378.
7. Bhide A, Shah PS and Acharya G. A simplified guide to randomized controlled trials. Acta Obstetricia et Gynecologica Scandinavica. 2018;97:380–387.
8. Moher D, Hopewell S, Schulz KF, et al. CONSORT 2010 explanation and elaboration: updated guidelines for reporting parallel group randomised trials. BMJ. 2010;340:c869.
9. Campbell MK, Piaggio G, Elbourne DR, Altman DG. CONSORT 2010 statement: extension to cluster randomised trials. BMJ. 2012;345:e5661.

10. Dumville JC, Hahn S, Miles JN, Torgerson DJ. The use of unequal randomisation ratios in clinical trials: a review. Contemporary Clinical Trials. 2006;27:1–12.

11. Ford I, Norrie J. Pragmatic trials. New England Journal of Medicine. 2016;375:454–63.

12. Loudon K, Treweek S, Sullivan F, Donnan P, Thorpe KE, Zwarenstein M. The PRECIS-2 tool: designing trials that are fit for purpose. BMJ. 2015;350:h2147.

13. RIGHT-2 Investigators: Bath PM, Scutt P, Anderson CS, Appleton JP, Berge E, Cala L, et al. Prehospital transdermal glyceryl trinitrate in patients with ultra-acute presumed stroke (RIGHT-2): an ambulance-based, randomised, sham-controlled, blinded, phase 3 trial. The Lancet. 2019;393:1009–20.

14. Perkins GD, Lall R, Quinn T, Deakin CD, Cooke MW, Horton J, et al. Mechanical versus manual chest compression for out-of-hospital cardiac arrest (PARAMEDIC): a pragmatic, cluster randomised controlled trial. The Lancet. 2015;385:947–55.

28

Experimental Studies Other than Randomised Controlled Trials

Andrew Fu Wah Ho, Audrey L Blewer and Marcus Ong

LEARNING OUTCOMES

1. Describe experimental clinical designs other than randomised controlled trials
2. Give examples of quasi-experimental and natural experiments

3. Recognise situations and scenarios where these designs are advantageous over randomised controlled trials
4. Describe the limitations of these designs as compared to randomised controlled trials

INTRODUCTION

Randomised controlled trials (RCT) are considered the gold standard of clinical research design, as they provide the highest internal validity for addressing questions of efficacy and effectiveness in healthcare, be it of a diagnostic tool, treatment, clinical pathway, strategy or policy. The random assignment in RCTs is key to the design strength. Without it, one cannot be certain that the difference in outcome between treatment arms is solely the effect of different treatment, or is distorted by confounders. However, an RCT is not always the best real-world strategy, due to practical and ethical difficulties.[1] As these situations are common in prehospital research (Fig 28.1), prehospital researchers should be aware of design techniques to handle such situations. However, an RCT is not always the best real-world strategy, due to practical an ethical difficulties, where there may be a need for experimental studies other than RCTs.

When RCTs are not feasible, investigators can adopt several alternative designs to address their research questions. First, they can modify the RCT design (see below) to circumvent these limitations while preserving randomised assignment. Second, they can use quasi-experimental designs, which are more commonly done. Third, where possible–and this is rare–they can take advantage of natural experiments. This chapter will be structured according to these three options, which are summarised in Table 28.1. These are not shortcuts for a well-designed RCT, which is rightfully the default design to answer interventional questions. While alternative methods can occasionally achieve high enough internal validity to be believable, many times they do not and become wasteful when an RCT is still needed. Therefore, the decision to deviate from an RCT design should be a deliberate one stemming from a pressing need to answer a research question when an RCT is impossible.

OPTION 1: MODIFICATIONS TO THE RCT DESIGN

Modifications can sometimes allow an RCT design where it is ordinarily not feasible. Here we give two examples.

Cohort Multiple RCT (cmRCT)

The cmRCT design by Relton and colleagues embeds an RCT into an existing cohort study.[2] Lengthy follow-up and high-quality outcome ascertainment are costly, but may already be done in existing registry studies. If the lack of funding or follow-up is the issue, the cmRCT allows for additional analyses at a lower cost. As an example, a trial investigating a new ambulance diversion policy for stroke could be designed with ambulances cluster-randomised to the new policy or current policy, and the outcome (such as timely receipt of thrombolysis or functional outcomes) ascertained using a national stroke registry.

Barriers	Lack of established clinical trial research infrastructure
	Lack of pilot trial data to robustly guide design and sample size calculations
	Prior understanding of the risk/benefit of the intervention and ethical considerations for assigning treatment
	Difficulty obtaining valid consent from severely ill patients (e.g. unconscious, agitated)
	Difficulty obtaining valid consent due to time and space constraints
	Some health systems require a doctor to be present to obtain consent
	Consent process may delay time-critical interventions
	Trial procedures encumber routine care which is already complex

Figure 28.1 Potential barriers to the conduct of rigorous RCT in the prehospital setting

TABLE 28.1	**Differences Between RCT, Quasi-Experiments and Natural Experiments**		
	Randomised Controlled Trial	**Quasi-Experiment**	**Natural Experiment**
Random assignment to treatment (A)	Yes. Researcher randomly assigns subjects to treatment groups (e.g. flipping a coin).	No. Researcher uses a non-random method to assign subjects to treatment groups (e.g. before-after, odd-even day, need, merit, risk).	Often (e.g. in 2008, Oregon used a lottery to ration Medicaid program among low-income, uninsured adults)
Control over treatment by researchers? (B)	Yes	Yes	No. Typically assigned by an external process outside the control of researcher.
True experiment (requires both A and B)	Yes	No	No
Initiated by	**Researcher**	**Researcher**	**Opportunistic**
Strength of causal inference if designed and conducted well	Typically high	Typically medium	Typically high. Caution: The term 'natural experiment' is sometimes used loosely. In these cases, causal inference can be much lower.
Example of designs	Clinical trial, community trial, pragmatic trial	Historical control, interrupted time series, simultaneous non-randomised control	

Modified Zelen's Design

This is a double-consent design to work around slow recruitment due to eligible patients being uncertain about treatment allocation.[3] Here, eligible patients are initially asked to consent only to randomisation and follow-up and then randomised. Specific consent for treatment is taken only if randomised to experimental treatment. If the latter consent is declined, the subject is given standard treatment and still followed up. The downside is that selection bias is introduced due to differential consent rate, and allocation concealment and blinding are violated.

Option 2: Quasi-Experimental Designs

In these interventional studies, treatment assignment is not random but rather is based on patient, clinician or researcher preference. They suffer from selection bias that needs to be controlled for in design and analysis. Quasi-experiments by definition require manipulation of the independent variable, but sometimes the data is already collected and one attempts to make the best of observational data to obtain insights about an intervention.

Historical Control (or Pretest–Posttest or Before–After Design)

Here, the average outcome of interest in a population is measured once before then once after a system-wide intervention is introduced. If the average posttest outcome is better than the average pretest outcome, then we might infer that the treatment was responsible for the improvement. While its simplicity is attractive, historical controls are ineffective-one cannot infer treatment effects with high certainty. We could be seeing

a baseline improving trend unaffected (or even restricted) by the treatment. The 'improvement' could also be due to a particularly bad month 'regressing to the mean'. The improvement could also be a result of many things other than the treatment, that change over time (often termed 'secular changes') or that influence the outcome or the quality of the outcome data.

Interrupted Time Series

This extends the pretest–posttest design by taking multiple measurements over time before and after a system-wide intervention is introduced. If the intervention is effective, it should cause an 'interruption' in the underlying trend. The advantage is clear when measurements are already collected routinely. However, it shares many limitations of the pretest–posttest design and is only marginally stronger causally. An example is a United Kingdom study evaluating a national quality improvement collaborative (QIC) on improvement in the delivery rate of care bundles in acute myocardial infarction and stroke patients. All English ambulance services were monitored between 2010 and 2012, during which a series of quality improvement initiatives were implemented. In the first report of this study, the authors used a simple historical control approach and found that care bundle performance for stroke in England improved from 83% to 96%, and concluded that the 'QIC led to significant improvements in ambulance stroke care'.[4] However, the excitement was tempered when a second report which treated the data as an interrupted time series, found that the improvement was no more than a secular trend (i.e. the improvement observed would likely have been seen even if the quality improvement program was not implemented) (see Fig 28.2).[5] These conflicting conclusions from

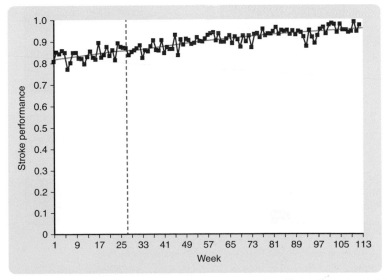

Figure 28.2 Using an interrupted time series approach to evaluate the effect of a national QIC on improvement in the delivery rate of care bundles and in stroke patients

the same data highlight the potential pitfall of quasi-experimental designs, where causal inferences are less robust.

Simultaneous Non-Randomised Control

This method applies a treatment to one group and compares its outcome improvement with a control group. There are many possible ways to select controls in a non-randomised fashion. For example, one could assign treatment based on means, preference and risk. We can then compare the average change in outcome among different treatment groups, thereby inferring efficacy. These non-random assignment methods introduce both selection bias and ascertainment bias (due to predictable and unmasked assignment). Statistical methods can reduce, but not eliminate these biases. An example is an emergency medical services (EMS) trial investigating endotracheal intubation (ETI) versus bag-valve-mask ventilation (BVM) in children.[6] Gausche and colleagues assigned paramedics to use ETI on odd-numbered days and BVM on even ones (Fig 28.3). The study found no evidence for the benefit of ETI in the out-of-hospital setting but did show a substantial increase in complications. Based on these findings, the Los Angeles and Orange County EMS agencies in California eliminated paediatric intubation from the scope of paramedic practice. In this case, selection bias is expected to be minimal as we do not expect patients to differ systematically on odd days and even days. However, the treatment and ascertainment biases from the loss of allocation concealment and blinding are limitations of the study.

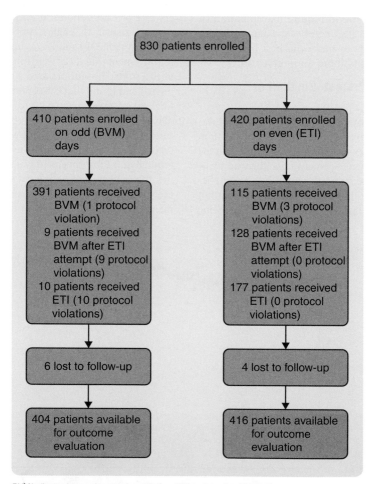

BVM indicates bag–valve–mask ventilation; *ETI*, endotracheal intubation.

Figure 28.3 Patient flow diagram used in a simultaneous non-randomised control trial of ETI versus bag–valve–mask ventilation

Statistical Approaches

In these non-randomised designs (including observational designs), one could analyse the data such that randomisation is mimicked. The common statistical techniques used to control for confounding are regression modelling (isolate the effect of exposure of interest while holding all confounders constant), propensity score matching (compare only cases and controls that have a similar likelihood of receiving treatment) and instrumental variable analysis.

Option 3: Natural Experiments

Natural experiments are 'true' experiments. They feature randomised assignment, but unlike RCTs, the randomisation occurs naturally, rather than being manipulated by investigators. Hence, they are *random* but not *controlled*. True natural experiments are rare (and indeed, the term is sometimes used loosely) and therefore their use is often opportunistic. Such natural experiments can provide robust causal inference at a fraction of the cost of an RCT, and should be leveraged when available. It requires the astute investigator to spot these opportunities and resourcefully capitalise on them.

CONCLUSION

In prehospital research, practical and ethical constraints sometimes necessitate interventional studies that are non-RCTs. Several alternatives are presented in this chapter. Their use needs to be coupled with a sound understanding of biases inherent in these designs, and their results are interpreted with caution. When used well, they can produce believable, practice-changing studies.

REVIEW QUESTIONS

1. Describe some experimental clinical designs other than RCT.
2. Explore a well-conducted non-RCT that has impacted paramedicine practice.
3. List some situations and scenarios where these designs are advantageous over RCT.
4. Describe the limitations of these designs as compared to RCT.

SUGGESTED FURTHER READING

Celentano DD, Szklo M, Gordis L. Using epidemiology to evaluate health services. In: Gordis epidemiology. 6th ed. Philadelphia: Elsevier; 2018.

Rothman KJ. Types of epidemiologic studies. In: Epidemiology: an introduction. 2nd ed. Oxford University Press; 2012.

West SG, Duan N, Pequegnat W, Gaist P, Des Jarlais, DC, Holtgrave D. et al. Alternatives to the randomized controlled trial. American Journal of Public Health. 2008;98:1359–66.

REFERENCES

1. Nichol G, Huszti E. Design and implementation of resuscitation research: special challenges and potential solutions. Resuscitation. 2007;73(3):337–46. Online. Available: https://doi.org/10.1016/j.resuscitation.2006.10.021.
2. Relton C, Torgerson D, O'Cathain A, Nicholl J. Rethinking pragmatic randomised controlled trials: Introducing the 'cohort multiple randomised controlled trial' design. BMJ. 2012;340:c1066. Online. Available: https://doi.org/10.1136/bmj.c1066.
3. Adamson J, Cockayne S, Puffer S, Torgerson DJ. Review of randomised trials using the post-randomised consent (Zelen's) design. Contemporary Clinical Trials. 2006;27(4):305–19. Online. Available: https://doi.org/10.1016/j.cct.2005.11.003.
4. Siriwardena AN, Shaw D, Essam N, Togher FJ, Davy Z, Spaight A, et al. The effect of a national quality improvement collaborative on prehospital care for acute myocardial infarction and stroke in England. Implementation Science. 2014;9:17. Online. Available: https://doi.org/10.1186/1748-5908-9-17.
5. Taljaard M, McKenzie JE, Ramsay CR, Grimshaw JM. The use of segmented regression in analysing interrupted time series studies: an example in pre-hospital ambulance care. Implementation Science. 2014;9(1):77. Online. Available: https://doi.org/10.1186/1748-5908-9-77.
6. Gausche M, Lewis RJ, Stratton SJ, Haynes BE, Gunter CS, Goodrich SM, et al. Effect of out-of-hospital pediatric endotracheal intubation on survival and neurological outcome: a controlled clinical trial. Journal of the American Medical Association. 2000;283(6):783. Online. Available: https://doi.org/10.1001/jama.283.6.783.

29

Data Collection Tools/Approaches for Quantitative Research

Nigel Rees

LEARNING OUTCOMES

- Introduction to data collection tools/approaches for quantitative research
- Introduction to the concepts of reliability and validity
- Exploring examples of data collection tools/approaches for quantitative research applied in out-of-hospital care studies

- Reflect on the barriers of data collection for quantitative research within the out-of-hospital environment

INTRODUCTION

Quantitative data collection approaches are versatile and powerful research methods and may include self-reporting tools, questionnaires, observation and biophysical measures. In this chapter, we discuss the importance of reliability and validity of data collection instruments, self-reported data tools as well as barriers to data collection. Finally, we present applied examples of data collection in out-of-hospital research.

RELIABILITY AND VALIDITY

When using quantitative data collection instruments, reliability and validity are essential. Reliability refers to the degree of consistency or accuracy with which an instrument measures the attribute it has been designed to measure, and unreliable instruments may result in incomplete or inaccurate data, limiting the ability to generalise the results to the larger population. Validity refers to the degree to which the instrument measures the phenomena of

interest in the first place or that it reflects the abstract construct being examined. The EQ-5D-5L is an example of one such validated instrument used by Fuller and colleagues in a pilot randomised controlled trial (RCT) of out-of-hospital continuous positive airway pressure (CPAP) for acute respiratory failure.[1]

SELF-REPORTED DATA COLLECTION TOOLS

A wide variety of self-reported data collection tools are also available. Surveys and questionnaires can be a quick way of collecting quantitative data from large samples of people, allowing comparisons between groups and subgroups and exploring differences and the reasons between them. Questionnaires may also be used to quantify specific information such as the Likert-rating scale which gives a specific range of choices from strongly agree to strongly disagree or always to never. However, such self-reported data collection may lack the depth of qualitative methods and the evaluative power of RCTs.

BARRIERS TO DATA COLLECTION IN THE OUT-OF-HOSPITAL SETTING

Conducting research in the out-of-hospital setting presents barriers unique to this environment, and data collection has been identified as a key barrier, especially when this context involves acutely sick or injured patients who cannot consent to treatment.[2] Barriers include gaining informed consent, lack of institutional support, rarity of the event (each paramedic treats only a few eligible patients), study enrolment and low study protocol compliance.[3-5] It has been argued that researchers with hospital-based backgrounds often lack such contextual knowledge when engaging in out-of-hospital research.[6,7] Early involvement and collaboration with out-of-hospital care professionals are therefore essential to developing and delivering effective out-of-hospital research, and data collection approaches should be carefully developed to reflect this context.[8]

APPLIED DATA COLLECTION IN OUT-OF-HOSPITAL CARE RESEARCH

Working with out-of-hospital care professionals, researchers have developed data collection methods, applying learning from previous trials to overcome such barriers. The PARAMEDIC2 trial reflects one such journey of out-of-hospital researchers to overcoming barriers to conduct complex research in this environment.[9] The PARAMEDIC2 trial built on the Prehospital Adrenaline for Cardiac Arrest (PACA) trial, which was the first RCT comparing adrenaline with placebo in out-of-hospital cardiac arrest and aimed to recruit 5000 patients but was stopped due to several factors, and just over 500 patients were recruited. The PARAMEDIC2 trial applied the learning from the PACA trial and included some of their investigators in the trial team.[9]

The PARAMEDIC2 trial was a randomised, double-blind trial involving 8014 patients with out-of-hospital cardiac arrest in the United Kingdom (UK). Paramedics at five National Health Service ambulance services administered either parenteral adrenaline (4015 patients) or saline placebo (3999 patients), along with standard care.[9] They conducted a 6-month internal pilot which included evaluation of whether their approach to data collection and follow-up worked effectively. The pilot ran seamlessly into the main trial and data from the pilot was included in the main study results.[10] The PARAMEDIC2 trial used many data collection approaches including recording survival to 30 days post-cardiac arrest, validated data collection instruments such as health-related quality of life at 3 and 6 months (SF12 and EQ-5D), modified Rankin Scale (mRS), incremental cost per quality-adjusted life-year (QALY), along with electronic data sets from sources such as the Intensive Care National Audit and Research Centre (ICNARC).[9]

Routinely collected information in medical records are often used to support research projects in out-of-hospital care aimed at the patient and societal benefit; some examples include the UK's Data Protection Act 2018 and the European Union's General Data Protection Regulation.[11,12] Consent forms and participant information sheets usually describe how data will be handled during a study, but occasionally researchers may use data without consent, which requires approval from an independent body. For example, in the UK the Confidentiality Advisory Group (CAG) is an independent national body that advises on the use of patient information. Large registries such as the UK's Out-of-Hospital Cardiac Arrest Outcomes Registry are examples of where such CAG advice has been applied.[13] Another examples may be the Victorian Ambulance Cardiac Arrest Registry (VACAR).

Snooks and colleagues reported on the pros and cons of using anonymised linked routine data to improve the efficiency of RCTs.[14] They report how regulatory processes, ethics, research and information governance permissions have caused a delay in each trial; however, inclusion rates have been much higher than is usual in RCTs and large trials have been achievable at a reasonable cost. Snooks and colleagues concluded that questions remain about differences between self-reported and routinely available outcomes; and between routine data outcomes collected prospectively and through the anonymised linked route.[14]

CONCLUSION

Data collection in out-of-hospital care research has its challenges. However, through careful selection of appropriate methods that are both reliable and validated, powerful and illuminating research can be conducted to improve patient care.

REVIEW QUESTIONS

1. Consider which data collection tools/approaches are appropriate for your research.
2. Is my data collection tools/approach valid and reliable? Why/why not?
3. What can you learn from other studies that have used data collection tools/approaches?

SUGGESTED FURTHER READING

Bruce N, Pope D, Stanistreet D. Quantitative methods for health research: a practical interactive guide to epidemiology and statistics paperback—abridged. 2nd ed. Wiley-Blackwell; 2018.

Greenhalgh TM, Bidewell J, Warland J, Lambros A, Crisp E. Understanding research methods for evidence-based practice in health. 2nd ed. Wiley; 2019.

REFERENCES

1. Fuller GW, Goodacre S, Keating S, Perkins G, Ward M, Rosser A, et al. The ACUTE (Ambulance CPAP: Use, Treatment effect and economics) feasibility study: a pilot randomised controlled trial of prehospital CPAP for acute respiratory failure. Pilot and Feasibility Studies. 18 June 2018;4(86). Online. Available: http://doi.org/10.1186/s40814-018-0281-9.

2. Lerner EB, Weik T, Edgerton EA. Research in prehospital care: overcoming the barriers to success, Prehospital Emergency Care. 2016;20(4):448–53. Online. Available: http://doi.org/10.3109/10903127.2014.980480.

3. Lockey DJ. Research questions in pre-hospital trauma care. PLoS Med. 2017;14:1002345.

4. Nichol G, Huszti E. Design and implementation of resuscitation research: special challenges and potential solutions. Resuscitation. 2007;73:337–46.

5. Ankolekar S, Parry R, Sprigg N, Niroshan Siriwardena A, Bath PMW. Views of paramedics on their role in an out-of-hospital ambulance-based trial in ultra-acute stroke: qualitative data from the Rapid Intervention With Glyceryl Trinitrate in Hypertensive Stroke Trial (RIGHT). Annals of Emergency Medicine. 1 December 2014;64(6):P640–8. Online. Available: https://pubmed.ncbi.nlm.nih.gov/24746844/.

6. Jensen JL, Bigham BL, Blanchard I, Dainty K, Socha D, Carter A, et al. The Canadian national EMS research agenda: a mixed methods consensus study. Canadian Journal of Emergency Medicine. 2013;15:73–82.

7. Leonard JC, Scharff DP, Koors V, Brooke Lerner E, Adelgais KM, Anders J, et al. A qualitative assessment of factors that influence emergency medical services partnerships in prehospital research. Academic Emergency Medicine. 2012;19:161–73.

8. Sayre MR, White LJ, Brown LH, McHenry SD. National EMS research agenda. Prehospital Emergency Care. 2002;6(sup3):S1–43.

9. Perkins DG, Ji C, Deakin CD, Quinn TM, Nolan JP, Scomparin C. Regan S, et al, for the PARAMEDIC2 Collaborators. Randomized trial of epinephrine in out-of-hospital cardiac arrest. New England Journal of Medicine. 18 July 2018. Online. Available: http://doi.org/10.1056/NEJMoa1806842.

10. Perkins GD, Quinn T, Deakin CD, Nolan JP, Lall R, Slowther AM, et al. Pre-hospital assessment of the role of adrenaline: measuring the effectiveness of drug administration in cardiac arrest (PARAMEDIC-2): trial protocol. Resuscitation. 2016;108:75–81. Online. Available: https://doi.org/10.1016/j.resuscitation.2016.08.029.

11. Data Protection Act 2018. United Kingdom; 2018. Online. Available: https://www.legislation.gov.uk/ukpga/2018/12/contents/enacted.

12. Guide to the General Data Protection Regulation. GOV.UK. 25 May 2018. Online. Available: https://www.gov.uk/government/publications/guide-to-the-general-data-protection-regulation.

13. Perkins DG, Brace-McDonnell SJ on behalf of the OHCAO Project Group. The UK Out of Hospital Cardiac Arrest Outcome (OHCAO) project. BMJ Open 2015;5:e008736. Online. Available: http://doi.org/10.1136/bmjopen-2015-008736.

14. Snooks H, Watkins A, Jones M, Khanom A, Jones J, Lyons RA. Pros and cons of using anonymised linked routine data to improve efficiency of randomised controlled trials in healthcare: experience in primary and emergency care. International Journal of Population Data Science. 2019;4(3). Online. Available: http://doi.org/10.23889/ijpds.v4i3.1250.

30

Types of Quantitative Data (Continuous, Categorical, Distributions, Skewness)

Yilin Ning, Nan Liu and Marcus Eng Hock Ong

LEARNING OUTCOMES

1. Identify different types of quantitative data
2. Understand the difference between data types
3. Detect skewed continuous data

INTRODUCTION

Data is a key part of any research study. For example, the Utstein style defines a comprehensive list of data to collect and report in an emergency care setting.[1] Depending on the nature of variables measured and the study aims, data may be quantified as different types. In this chapter, we group quantitative data into two general classes (continuous and categorical), describe their key statistical properties and discuss how these properties may affect subsequent analyses.

CONTINUOUS DATA

Continuous data refers to data that can be 'measured', and can take any value within a range. For example, age or call-response intervals are continuous data. Research questions asked about continuous data usually concern changes in numerical values; for example, the increased risk of death per unattended minute after cardiac arrest.

CATEGORICAL DATA

In contrast, categorical data is data that is divided into groups. For example, when studying age, the data can be divided into 5-year or 10-year age groups rather than be analysed as a continuous variable.

Categorical data can be ordinal or nominal. For example, age groups have a natural ordering, and so is considered ordinal data. Another example of ordinal data is the Australasian Triage Scale which uses five categories to indicate the clinical urgency for emergency patients, with categories 1 to 5 ordered in a decreasing level of urgency.[2] Some categorical data do not have any informative ordering; for example, gender (male or female) or bystander CPR (yes, no or unknown). Such categorical data is nominal.

Research questions concerning categorical data usually test for differences between categories. For example, is the chance of receiving bystander CPR higher for males or females? For ordinal data, it is also relevant to test for trend when the ordinal level increases. For example, does the risk of cardiac arrest increase for higher age groups?

DATA DISTRIBUTION

The probability distribution quantifies how likely (or unlikely) it is to observe a given value in the data, which forms the basis for statistical inference. The distribution of categorical data (both nominal and ordinal) is simply described by the total number of observations and the proportion of observations in each category. For continuous data, the most encountered probability distribution is the normal distribution, which assumes that the data is symmetrically distributed around a mean (i.e. the average value). Figure 30.1 visually illustrates a normal distribution. The spread of data is quantified by the standard deviation, and approximately 95% of data is within two standard deviations from the mean, corresponding to the area shaded in grey in Figure 30.1.

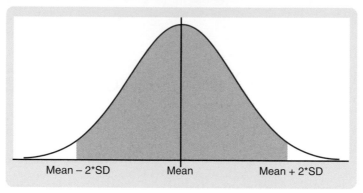

Figure 30.1 An example of a normal distribution. SD: standard deviation

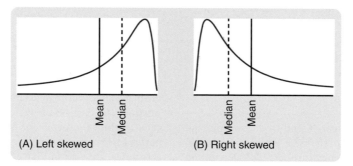

Figure 30.2 Examples of skewed distributions

SKEWNESS

Statistical analysis of continuous data often relies on the assumption that the data is normally (or at least symmetrically) distributed. Distribution is symmetric when the mathematical mean coincides with the median (i.e. the value that is lying at the midpoint of a frequency distribution). Figure 30.2A shows a distribution that is skewed to the left, where the left tail is longer than the right tail, and the median is larger than the mean. A right-skewed distribution such as that shown in Figure 30.2B has a longer right tail and a median smaller than the mean.

EXAMPLE USING CARDIAC ARREST DATA

Using the age of patients in an out-of-hospital cardiac arrest registry, we illustrate how to assess the skewness of continuous data in practice.

Compare Mean and Median

The mean age is 69.4 years and the median is 74.0 years, suggesting the distribution may be left-skewed.

Visual Assessment Using a Histogram

The distribution of continuous data can be visually assessed using a histogram (see Fig 30.3), which visualises the number of observations in each predefined interval. The longer left tail of the distribution also suggests left skewness.

CORRECT IDENTIFICATION OF DATA TYPES

Different types of data have various properties that need to be handled using appropriate statistical methods. This seemingly trivial step can sometimes be controversial.

For example, Quality of Life (QoL) data quantifies the wellbeing of patients using numeric scores that often range from 0 to 100. The European Quality of Life–5 Dimensions

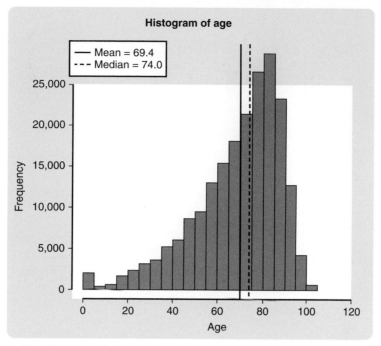

Figure 30.3 Histogram of the age of patients who had an out-of-hospital cardiac arrest

(EQ-5D) is used in the Pan-Asian Resuscitation Outcomes Study (PAROS) to quantify the overall health status of cardiac arrest survivors.[3] Many researchers treat QoL data as a continuous variable despite an important limitation: the same numerical change in the scores (e.g. a 10-point increase in the scores from 0 to 10 or from 90 to 100) does not necessarily correspond to the same change in patients' wellbeing. QoL data is often highly skewed, which also affects the choice of analytical approaches.[4] Hence, it is important to understand the definition and basic properties of data (e.g. is the data truly continuous and how is it distributed), before performing a statistical analysis.

CONCLUSION

In this chapter, we described two types of quantitative data, continuous and categorical, that are commonly encountered

in paramedic research. Although both types of data may be represented using numeric values and hence appear to be similar (e.g. age in years and an ordinal QoL variable ranging from 0 to 100), these variables convey different types of information and have different statistical properties that need to be handled using different analytical methods. Hence, correct identification of data types is essential in quantitative research.

REVIEW QUESTIONS

1. What are the data types described in this chapter?
2. What is the difference between nominal and ordinal data?
3. The histogram below shows the distribution of the length of stay (LOS) of a group of patients in the emergency department (ED). Is the distribution of ED LOS skewed, and if yes, is it skewed to the left or to the right?

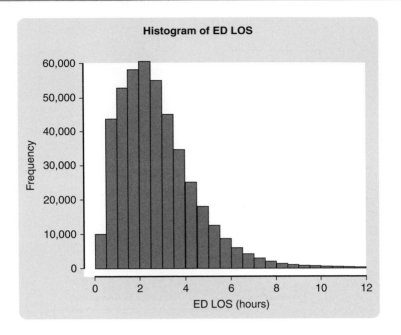

Histogram of ED LOS

REFERENCES

1. Otto Q, Nolan JP, Chamberlain DA, Cummins RO, Soar J. Utstein Style for emergency care—the first 30 years. Resuscitation. 2021;163:16–25.
2. Australian College for Emergency Medicine. Triage. n.d. Online. Available: https://acem.org.au/Content-Sources/Advancing-Emergency-Medicine/Better-Outcomes-for-Patients/Triage.
3. Ong MEH, Shin S Do, Tanaka H, Ma MH-M, Khruekarnchana P, Hisamuddin N, et al. Pan-Asian Resuscitation Outcomes Study (PAROS): rationale, methodology and implementation. Academic Emergency Medicine. 2011;18(8): 890–7.
4. Fayers PM, Machin D. Quality of life: the assessment, analysis and interpretation of patient-reported outcomes. 2nd ed. Chichester, UK: John Wiley & Sons, Ltd; 2007.

31

Descriptive Statistics, Missing Data and Testing Assumptions

Yu-Tung Chang

LEARNING OUTCOMES

1. Understand when and how to implement descriptive statistical analysis to your data
2. Understand the approaches to managing missing data
3. Understand the importance of assumptions testing

DESCRIPTIVE STATISTICS

DEFINITION

Descriptive statistics can be defined as an analytical approach to describing the data at your disposal.[1] This approach aims to summarise and extract data information and characteristics into certain numbers, tables or graphs.

INTRODUCTION

Before we start to adopt advanced statistical methods, it is important to conduct descriptive statistics analysis to have a basic understanding of what your data looks like.

Missing data or missing values occur when we collect incomplete records or observations in the study process.[1,2] Sometimes it is unavoidable. Missing data can be caused by random situations (unexpected) or research design problems. For example, a participant forgets to respond to questions in a questionnaire, or a certain variable is too difficult to be observed. There are three types of missing values: missing completely at random (MCAR), missing at random (MAR) or not missing at random (NMAR).[1,2]

Statistical testing is an important step in data analysis. The results of the testing are the basis of a study's conclusion. When we conduct a study, we have to identify the research questions and make assumptions (expected answers) of this study. For testing the research assumptions, we have to collect certain data that may provide useful information to support the assumptions. Researchers will have to select statistical testing methods according to data types, data structures and these assumptions.[1,2]

There may be many variables in the data we collect. For example, if we collect 30 days of vital signs from a patient record, this may consist of many variables like blood pressure, heart rate and oxygen saturation. Each variable, such as blood pressure, consists of 30 blood pressure values. What do the 30 records of blood pressure tell us? There are a few methods to describe the data, such as measures of location, spread and data presentation.

The impact of missing data on study results can be minor or major. If the number of missing values accounts for a very low proportion of the total number of observations, then we can try to ignore these missing observations. However, it is difficult to determine the exact proportion of missing values that could impact the results.[1,2] Researchers have to evaluate and test the impact when we keep or remove the observations with missing values based on the importance of the variables with missing values.[1,2]

In statistics, the assumption of the above example can be written in two hypotheses. The first hypothesis, the so-called 'null hypothesis' (H_0), is an assumption that assumes the observed sample variable has no difference between the same variable of population or other comparison groups.[1,2] The second hypothesis, the 'alternative hypothesis' (H_1), is an assumption that assumes the observed sample variable has differences between the same variable of population or another comparison group.[1,2]

EXAMPLES

Measures of location are also known to measure the central tendency of the data. The most common use of measures of location are arithmetic mean, median and mode.[1] Those measures represent and describe the location where most of the data are centrally distributed.[1] The reason we measure the location of data is to make sure that the sample data we collected has a similar distribution (or data shape) to our target population.[1] The degree of difference between the location of sample and target population data can be used to test the statistical significance in many statistical methods, such as the t-test.[1]

Measures of spread aim to measure the variance between each data point or the distance between each data point and the arithmetic mean of the data.[1] The most common use of measures are range, variance and standard deviation. If the result of this measure is high, the data points are far away from each other on average.[1] The result of spread measurement can be also used to test the statistical significance in many statistical methods, such as F-test in ANOVA and linear regression.[1–3]

Data presentations, such as tables, figures and charts, are often used by researchers to demonstrate the characteristics of the data. These methods can present frequency, percentage, tendency and cross-reference numbers. The most common data presentation methods are histograms, diagrams, pie charts and contingency tables.[1–4]

There are three methods to deal with missing values: 1. complete case analysis, where only those cases with complete data and no missing values are included; 2. available data analysis, where all collected data is included; and 3. imputation methods, which adapt mathematical approaches to estimate the missing values. In MCAR situations, you can directly analyse the collected data without processing the missing values. However, the second and third methods are better. If the type of missing value is missing at random, the multiple imputation method is recommended.[1,3]

For example, we may assume that participants in group A have a higher blood pressure value than those in group B. We may choose a t-test to test whether the average blood pressure values between the two groups have statistical differences or not. In this case, the null hypothesis is 'The blood pressure values are no different between group A and group B'. The alternative hypothesis is 'The blood pressure values are different between group A and group B'.[1]

CONCLUSION

Descriptive statistics is the first step in exploring data. We consider adapting statistical testing methods based on the result of descriptive statistical analysis. There are numerous software programs (e.g. SPSS, Stata, R) that can assist us to complete descriptive statistical analysis easily.

Missing data can be seen as a technique to manage your research data. There are many approaches to deal with missing data in statistical or non-statistical bases. However, approaches to managing missing data are unable to create the same effect as the real data from the population. Therefore, we suggest designing and rigorously collecting data to avoid the occurrence of missing data.

When you identify the research questions, you can also write the null and alternative hypotheses for each question. This step will be essential for researchers to determine the research objective and choose appropriate statistics testing methods.

REVIEW QUESTIONS

1. Review the Out-of-Hospital Cardiac (OHCA) Arrest Utstein data from your region in the recent 5 years. How will you describe the 5-year data?
2. Imagine you are collecting OHCA data for research purposes and you find out there are few data missing. How will you deal with this situation? How will you maintain the balance between clinical and statistical significance?
3. What research questions would you like to explore using Utstein data?

SUGGESTED FURTHER READING

Rosner B. Fundamentals of biostatistics. 6th ed. US: Duxbury Press; 2005.

Victorian Ambulance Cardiac Arrest Registry (VACAR). VACAR 2019–2020 Annual Report. Ambulance Victoria; 2020. Online. Available: https://www.ambulance.vic.gov.au/wp-content/uploads/2021/02/VACAR-Annual-Report-2019-2020_FINAL_Feb2021.pdf

REFERENCES

1. Rosner B. Fundamentals of biostatistics. 6th ed. US: Duxbury Press; 2005.
2. Norman G, Streiner DL, Streiner D. Biostatistics: the bare essentials. 3rd ed. US: PMPH USA; 2008.
3. Gentleman R, Hornik K, Parmigiani G. Biostatistics with R: an introduction to statistics through biological data. US: Springer; 2012.
4. Hoffman T, Bennett S, Del Mar C. Evidence-based practice across the health professions. 3rd ed. Australia: Elsevier; 2017.

32

Confidence Intervals, *p*-values, Effect Size and Statistical Significance

Alexander Olaussen and Gerard O'Reilly

LEARNING OUTCOMES

1. Be able to define confidence intervals, *p*-values and effect size
2. Gain an appreciation for the parameters included in the calculation of *p*-values
3. Discuss the meaning of statistical significance and compare it to clinical significance

DEFINITIONS

- Confidence intervals: The range of potential effect sizes.
- *p*-value: The probability of observing an equal or more extreme result given the null hypothesis is true (i.e. assuming no difference between groups).
- Effect size: The magnitude of the measure of association or difference.
- Statistical significance: The confidence in the effect being real (i.e. not occurring by chance).

INTRODUCTION

When we compare two things, how can we tell if that difference is likely to be true or just random variation between the samples, and how confident are we in our conclusion about this? These questions form the foundation for common statistical concepts such as *p*-values and confidence intervals covered in this chapter. The following concepts are described in a variety of ways across the literature and it has been demonstrated that 89% of textbooks incorrectly define or explain statistical significance—so be cautious.[1]

Steps in Hypothesis Testing

Before discussing *p*-values and statistical significance, it is worth revising the steps in hypothesis testing—which to the novice researcher can seem somewhat counterintuitive. Let's say we hypothesise that ketamine is effective in reducing the respiratory rate (RR) in asthma. We would do the following steps in statistical methods. First, we would create our null hypothesis (H0), which is that there is no difference in the RR between the patients given ketamine and those that are given placebo (or something else). As the ketamine may both increase and decrease the RR, we should choose a two-tailed test (because we are agnostic as to which direction the impact of ketamine may be). We would then collect data on patients who received and did not receive ketamine (ideally in a randomised controlled trial, but the statistics would be the same for observational studies). We would decide our significance level (i.e. alpha) below which we will reject the H0 (thus making our initial or alternate hypothesis true). The alpha for the vast majority of articles is arbitrarily and conventionally set at 5% or 0.05. This means that we accept a 1 in 20 probability that what we observe may be due to chance.

Confidence Intervals

Let's say we have 200 patients in our ketamine trial. When reporting the age of the cohort, we would first look at a histogram of the age and determine if that data is distributed normally (i.e. parametric) or skewed to one side (i.e. non-parametric) (see Figure 32.1).

For parametric distributions (of continuous data) we should report the mean (i.e. the point estimate) and the standard deviation.

Now, for the 95% confidence interval (CI) of the difference in mean age (i.e. the effect size or measure of

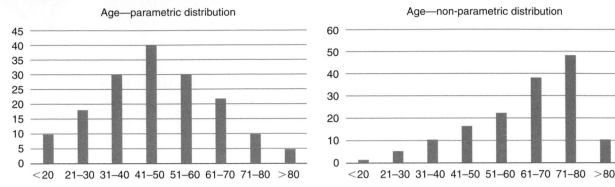

Figure 32.1 Examples of histograms showing parametric and non-parametric (i.e. skewed data)

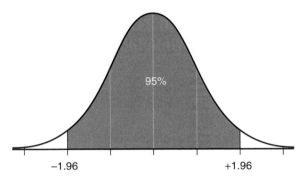

Figure 32.2 In normal distribution, 95% of the observations lie within 2 (or more accurately, 1.96) standard deviations of the mean

$$variance = S^2 = \sigma^2 = \frac{\Sigma(X_i - X_{mean})^2}{n-1}$$

Now that we have the variance, we can calculate the t statistic, which is worked out as follows:

$$t = \frac{X_{mean} - Y_{mean}}{\sqrt{\frac{(nx-1)\,S^2x + (ny-1)S^2y}{nx + ny - 2}} \times \sqrt{(\frac{1}{nx} + \frac{1}{ny})}}$$

Where X_{mean} and Y_{mean} are the mean (RRs) in the ketamine group and the non-ketamine group, respectively; nx and ny is the number of patients in each of those two groups; and S^2x and S^2y is the variance in each group. The resultant t-value can then be located in a 't-test table' and the p-value revealed.

Although the above formulae may appear daunting, be reassured by the fact that very few researchers know these automatically. The reason for presenting the formulae here is to highlight the importance of sample size. With increasing sample size, the variance will shrink and thus be producing statistically significant p-values more often. This is particularly relevant in the setting of large volumes of data (i.e. big data) and repeated testing (e.g. with artificial intelligence). Since there is nothing in this world that is identical to another thing—even two snowflakes—the only relevant question then is clinical relevance.[3]

p-values have attracted much debate, emotions and misuse in the medical literature.[4] In 2016, the American Statistical Association published six guiding principles regarding the reporting of p-values to alleviate some of the confusion and misuses.[5]

1. p-values can indicate how incompatible the data are with a specified statistical model.
2. p-values do <u>not</u> measure the probability that the studied hypothesis is true, or the probability that the data were produced by random chance alone.

association between the two groups)—which is 1.96 standard deviations (of the effect size) either side of the calculated difference in mean age (also named as the '1.96 standard errors of the difference in means')—describes a range within which 95% of the real (population) effect size will lie (e.g. for a difference in mean age of xx, the 95%CI = a difference in mean age between xx and xx years). See Figure 32.2.

p-value

The p-value can be defined as follows: 'the p-value is the probability of obtaining our results, or something more extreme, if the null hypothesis is true'.[2] While p-values are calculated on statistical software, it is valuable to understand the formulas which underpins them. First, consider the variance—a measure of spread which is calculated by considering how far away from the mean each observation is. If the spread of RR observations in either group (ketamine or placebo) is small in either direction, then the variance would be small, but if the spread of RR observations is large, then the variance is large.

3. Scientific conclusions and business or policy decisions should **not** be based only on whether a *p*-value passes a specific threshold.
4. Proper inference requires full reporting and transparency.
5. A *p*-value, or statistical significance, does not measure the size of an effect or the importance of a result.
6. By itself, a *p*-value does not provide a good measure of evidence regarding a model or hypothesis.

Statistical Significance Versus Clinical Significance

When considering the word significance, synonyms such as important and meaningful come to mind. The concept of clinical significance or clinical importance—but not statistical significance—deals with these concepts. For instance, if drug A lowers the blood pressure by 2 mmHg more than drug B (i.e. the effect size is a difference in mean systolic blood pressure of 2 mmHg), that is probably not clinically meaningful or significant, although with enough patient data this difference would be reported as statistically significant. On the other hand, statistical significance deals with whether or not the observed difference between drug A and drug B are likely to have arisen by chance or whether the difference is truly present. As mentioned previously—since nothing is identical—the latter will always be the case.

EXAMPLES

The PARAMEDIC2 trial, which compared adrenaline/epinephrine to placebo in cardiac arrest, reported that 'in the epinephrine group, 130 patients (3.2%) were alive at 30 days, as compared with 94 patients (2.4%) in the placebo group (unadjusted odds ratio for survival, 1.39; 95% confidence interval [CI], 1.06 to 1.82; $p = 0.02$)'.[6]

This means that if we repeated the trial many times, the odds ratio (i.e. the effect size) of adrenaline/epinephrine would end up being somewhere between 1.06 and 1.82, 95% of the time. Another acceptable way of interpreting this is that we are 95% certain that the true (i.e. population) results lie somewhere between 1.06 (the lower confidence limit) and 1.82 (the upper confidence limit). The *p*-value of 0.02 tells us the result is statistically significant (i.e. less than 5% chance of obtaining this result by chance). We can also conclude that the result (odds ratio) is statistically significant because the CI did not cross one.

CONCLUSION

Null-hypothesis significance testing is a critical component of research. *p*-values and CIs provide suggestions as to whether or not we should reject the null hypothesis (i.e. whether or not what we have observed is true or not). If the probability of obtaining the result (or something even more extreme) is less than our pre-determined significance level (typically 0.05, or 5%), then we reject the null hypothesis and conclude there is evidence to support the alternative hypothesis.

REVIEW QUESTIONS

1. Consider the difference between statistical and clinical significance. Think of examples that may be statistically significant but not clinically significant. And conversely, is it possible to have clinically significant findings that are not statistically significant?
2. Given the fact that an increasing sample size decreases the variance and tightens the confidence interval, what implications does this carry in terms of calculating and interpreting statistical significance for small and large studies?
3. How do you decide what a clinically significant change is?

SUGGESTED FURTHER READING

Ioannidis JPA. Why most published research findings are false. PLOS Medicine. 2005;2(8):e124.
Kirkwood B. Sterne J. Essentials of Medical Statistics, 2nd ed. Oxford: Blackwell Publishing; 2003.
Wasserstein RL, Lazar NA. The ASA Statement on p-Values: Context, Process, and Purpose. The American Statistician. 2016;70(2):129–33.

REFERENCES

1. Cassidy SA, Dimova R, Giguère B, Spence JR, Stanley DJ. Failing grade: 89% of introduction-to-psychology textbooks that define or explain statistical significance do so incorrectly. Advances in Methods and Practices in Psychological Science. 2019;2(3):233–9.
2. Petrie A, Sabin C. Medical statistics at a glance. 3rd ed. Singapore: Wiley-Blackwell; 2009.
3. Krevat E, Tucek J, Ganger GR, editors. Disks are like snowflakes: no two are alike. HotOS; 2011.
4. Olaussen A, Abetz J, Qin KR, Mitra B, O'Reilly G. Misleading medical literature: an observational study. Emerg Med Australas. 2021.
5. Wasserstein RL, Lazar NA. The ASA Statement on p-Values: Context, Process, and Purpose. The American Statistician. 2016;70(2):129–33.
6. Perkins GD, Ji C, Deakin CD, et al. A randomized trial of epinephrine in out-of-hospital cardiac arrest. New England Journal of Medicine. 2018;379(8):711–21.
7. Ioannidis JPA. Why most published research findings are false. PLOS Medicine. 2005;2(8):e124.

33

Inferential Statistics: T-Tests, Regression Analysis and Adjustments (Mediation Versus Moderation)

Alaa Oteir

LEARNING OUTCOMES

1. Identify the tests used to compare means between two independent groups
2. Identify the tests used to compare means between two dependent groups
3. Identify the non-parametric equivalent tests
4. Understand the importance and aim of using simple linear and multiple linear regression
5. Understand the importance and aim of using simple logistic regression
6. Identify and understand the assumptions related to linear regression
7. Understand how to report the finding of linear and logistic regression

INTRODUCTION

In this chapter, we discuss when to use t-tests, linear regression and logistic regression. We will also learn the importance and aim of using these tests and highlight how to report the findings appropriately.

T-TESTS

A t-test aims to examine the difference between the means of a dependent variable between independent groups.[1] There are two types of t-test, including the independent sample t-test (student's t-test) and the dependent sample t-test or paired t-test.[1,2] The independent samples t-test examines the difference in means between two independent groups, given that the variable is a continuous variable and data are normally distributed. For example, we can compare the systolic blood pressure or heart rate between males and females or who received a specific intervention and did not. On the other hand, we can use a dependent t-test when comparing the systolic blood pressure

TABLE 33.1 Parametric and its Equivalent Non-Parametric Tests

Two Samples*	Parametric	Non-Parametric
Independent	Student's t-test	Mann–Whitney U test
Dependent	Paired sample t-test	Wilcoxon signed-rank test

*Continuous variables

before and after a particular intervention (or at two different time points) for the same group of participants.

In case the data are non-parametric (not normally distributed, usually sample size less than 30), then the equivalent non-parametric tests are as illustrated in Table 33.1.

REGRESSION ANALYSES

Regression analysis is used to predict or examine the nature of the association between two variables. Although there are different types of regression, in this chapter we will discuss the most commonly used ones: linear regression and logistic regression. Then we will describe simple/binary and multiple/multivariate regression.

LINEAR REGRESSION

Linear regression examines the relationships between a continuous outcome (dependent) variable and one or more independent/predictor (continuous or categorical) variables. This represents how much the independent variable can explain the variable in the outcome variable, using R^2. Also, it provides the correlation between these variables.

In simple linear regression, we examine the relationship between a single predictor (independent) variable and an outcome variable. Multivariate linear regression examines how much variance in the outcome variable can be explained by multiple predictors. It also aims to produce a model that best predicts the actual outcome value.

Some assumptions must be met in the linear regression, including:

- a linear relationship between the outcome variable and the predictor variables
- multivariate normality—that the residuals are normally distributed
- no multicollinearity—that the predictor variables are not highly correlated with each other; this can be checked using the variance inflation factor (VIF) values (a VIF $\geq$ 10 means there is multicollinearity)
- that observations be independent of one another. The following can be included in the report.
1. The R^2 (the square or correlation coefficient) represents the variance in the outcome.
2. The F statistics and its p-value indicate whether the model is significant and successful.
3. The beta coefficient for the significant predictors, p-value and/or the 95% CI.

LOGISTIC REGRESSION

Logistic regression examines the likelihood of a dependent variable occurrence based on one or more predictor variables. In binary logistic regression, the outcome has two categories (yes or no; high or low; survived or not survived). The test examines the relationship with one predictor variable (e.g. smoking status, age, sex; or preexisting conditions) or multiple predictors. This relationship is presented as an odds ratio (OR), which can be below one (less likely to occur or has a protective effect), greater than one (more likely to occur) or the value of one (no change/no difference).

Some assumptions must be met in the logistic regression, including:

- a linear relationship between the predictor and the log of the outcome variable
- no multicollinearity
- that observations should be independent of each other. The following can be included in the report:[2]
- R^2 stating the amount of variance explained
- Hosmer and Lemeshow's goodness of fit (other measures also available)
- the predictors that successfully predicted the outcomes
- the odds ratio of the predicting variables and its p-value and/or 95% CI.

GENERAL NOTES

It should be noted that there are different methods of data entry in multiple linear regression. The choice of these methods depends on the nature research question, type of data, author's choice and/or statistical software in use.

EXAMPLES

Example 1

Is there a difference in the levels measured by the depression, anxiety and stress scale (DASS) between males and female frontline responders who deal with COVID-19 patients?

Required Tests

If outcomes (DASS levels) are normally distributed, an independent t-test (student t-test) is appropriate to compare the means between males and females. However, if these outcomes were not normally distributed (or the sample size is less than 30), then medians are compared using the Mann–Whitney U test.

If the scores were taken at two different time points (e.g. at the beginning of the pandemic and 6 months/1 year after) for the same participants, then a paired-test or Wilcoxon signed-rank test is appropriate.

Example 2

What are the predictor(s) of DASS levels among frontline responders who deal with COVID-19 patients?

Each outcome measure is a continuous variable, meaning that linear regression analysis is appropriate to identify the predictors here. However, if the researchers decided to categorise the DASS scores into normal and abnormal levels, a logistic regression analysis would be the appropriate test to examine the relationship between the different factors and these outcome measures.

CONCLUSION

In this chapter, we discussed that an independent t-test is used to compare the means of two independent groups, whereas a dependent or paired t-test compares the mean of the same groups at two different time points (e.g. before and after an intervention). We also learned that the Mann–Whitney U test and Wilcoxon signed-rank test are the non-parametric equivalents to students' t-test and paired t-test, respectively. Furthermore, we discussed that regression is used to examine the relationship between an outcome variable and an independent/predictor variable(s). Linear regression is used when we have a continuous outcome, whereas binary logistic regression analysis is used when we have categorical (two categories) outcome variables. Finally, several assumptions must be met to confirm the appropriateness of these regression tests, and recommendations on how to report the findings were provided.

REVIEW QUESTIONS

1. Which test should you choose when comparing the means of a certain measure:
   a. between two independent groups
   b. twice for the same group at two timepoints?
2. What are the equivalent non-parametric tests for the t-test?
3. What test should be used to examine the relationship between a predictor and a continuous outcome variable?
4. What test should be used to examine the relationship between a predictor and a categorical (binary) outcome variable?
5. What value should be reported in regression analysis?
6. What are the assumptions that must be met in the regression analysis?

SUGGESTED FURTHER READING

Hamilton LC. Statistics with Stata: version 12. Cengage Learning, 2012.
Mayers A. Introduction to statistics and SPSS in psychology. Pearson Education; 2013.
Pallant J. Survival manual. A step by step guide to data analysis using IBM SPSS. 7th ed. Routledge; 2020.
Seber GA, Lee AJ. Linear regression analysis. John Wiley & Sons; 2012.

REFERENCES

1. Kim TK. T test as a parametric statistic. Korean Journal of Anesthesiology. 2015;68(6):540.
2. Mayers A. Introduction to statistics and SPSS in psychology. Pearson Education; 2013.

34

An Introduction to Survival Analysis

Gerard M O'Reilly

LEARNING OUTCOMES

1. Develop a basic understanding of the role of survival analysis

2. Have an introductory familiarity with the tools of survival analysis

DEFINITION

Survival analysis is the branch of data analysis methods dealing with 'time-to-event' data. The term 'survival time' refers to the length of time from the time of a fixed starting point (e.g. time of arrival of the ambulance at scene) to the time point at which an event occurs. An 'event' can be anything of research interest, for which the 'time-to' is measured. Examples of an 'event' relevant to prehospital emergency care include hospital arrival and initiation of specific interventions.

INTRODUCTION

Quality indicators for prehospital emergency care include measures of the 'time-to' various interventions, including time at scene, time to hospital and time to various specific interventions (e.g. analgesia, endotracheal intubation, initiation of cardiopulmonary resuscitation). To increase the validity of analyses of 'time-to-event' data, it is important to have at least an introductory understanding of the role and tools of survival analysis methods.

For many analyses where 'time-to-event' is of research interest, simpler methods can be used as follows.

1. If *all* (or almost all) subjects are followed up until the occurrence of the event, the mean (of survival times or log-transformed survival times as the data is often skewed) or median (of the survival times) in each group can be used as a summary measure of central tendency. Then the measure of association used to compare two groups would be the difference in mean (or equivalent for log-transformed survival time) or median survival time (time-to-event) between those two groups.

2. If the focus of the research question is *not* the distribution of the survival *time* itself but the *proportion* of subjects having the event by a predefined endpoint, then the proportion (of subjects) for whom the event of research interest (e.g. death, return of spontaneous circulation) occurred within a specified timeframe (e.g. 30 minutes following ambulance arrival) can be used as the measure of central tendency. Then the measure of association used to compare the two groups would be the difference in proportions, risk ratio or odds ratio across the two groups.

However, if the focus of the research question is the distribution of the survival *time* itself (i.e. not as for option 2, above, the *proportion* having the event by a predefined endpoint) **but** some subjects do not have the event (i.e. they are 'censored') during the study period (i.e. not option 1, above, when all, or almost all subjects have the event), then survival analysis methods are required. Censoring or censored data is when subjects do not reach the event of interest during the study period (e.g. where return of spontaneous circulation [ROSC]) is the predefined 'event', ROSC does not occur or the patient is declared dead before arrival at hospital). For censored subjects, their survival time (time-to-event) is greater than the time period for which they are in the study (e.g. they never achieve ROSC before hospital arrival).

TOOLS FOR SURVIVAL ANALYSIS

There are two main approaches to analysing survival data. The first of these (the survival curve) applies to all survival analyses; the application of the second approach (the hazard ratio) depends on meeting criteria for the proportional hazards assumption.

1. Survival Curve

The survival curve, generated using estimations derived by the Kaplan–Meier method, summarises graphically the probability of surviving beyond time 't', with t on the X-axis and survival probability (beyond time = t) on the Y-axis (see Figure 34.1). The units of time, denoted by t, will be relatively small compared to the study period (e.g. minutes for prehospital emergency care research).

The statistical measure for comparing the survival curves (i.e. the entire survival experience) between groups is known as the log-rank test, which generates a p-value against the chi-square distribution. The null hypothesis for this test is that the survival (time-to-event) experience is the same for the different exposure groups.

It is important to note that the survival curve and its derived log-rank test do not provide a numerical estimate for the difference in survival (i.e. a numerical summary measure of association or effect size) between the exposure groups.[1–3]

2. Hazard Ratio

Hazard is the instantaneous risk of death (i.e. the event occurring) given alive (i.e. the event not yet occurring) at time = t. While the survival curve summaries *risk* (of *not*

having the event) over a preceding *period* of time, the hazard function summarises the instantaneous risk (of *having* the event) at a point in time. Hazard is a *rate*, and the hazard rate varies over time.

The hazard ratio is the ratio of hazard rates in two groups. It provides another way (to the visualisation of the survival curves) of comparing survival experience between two groups. Whereas the survival curves generate a test of statistical significance (confidence) but no numerical summary measure of association or comparison, the hazard ratio is a numerical summary measure of association for comparing two groups. Furthermore, the hazard ratio can also generate the equivalent of the log-rank test of statistical confidence (in the null hypothesis of no difference between hazard functions). Finally, the hazard ratio allows for the testing for the presence of confounding and effect modification, using regression methods, known as the Cox proportional hazards regression methods.

It is important to note that the hazard ratio and the corresponding Cox proportional hazards regression methods depend on the hazard ratio being constant. That is, while the hazard rates will vary with time, the relationship of these hazard rates (described by the hazard ratio) needs to remain constant for this to be a valid analysis tool. There are a variety of methods that are used to check that the proportion hazards assumption is valid, both graphical and statistical.[1–3]

CONCLUSION

A basic understanding of the tools used for survival analysis is important to the 'time-to' focused domain of prehospital

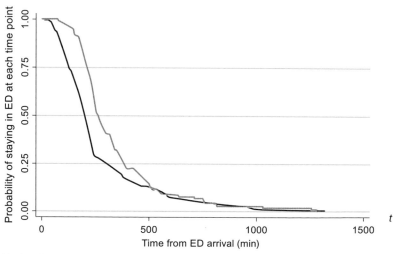

Figure 34.1 Kaplan–Meier plot for probability of continuing to stay in ED. Log-rank test for equality of survivor functions: $p = 0.001$. (——) No isolation in ED; (——) Isolation in ED (Source: O'Reilly GM et al. Impact of patient isolation on emergency department length of stay: a retrospective cohort study using the Registry for Emergency Care. Emergency Medicine Australasia. 2020; 32(6): 1034-1039.)

emergency care research. If outcome data is complete or the focus is on the proportion of subjects reaching the 'event' during the study period, then simple methods can be employed. But for a more time-focused analysis, survival curves and the log-rank test are important tools, with the added utilisation of the hazard ratio and Cox regression methods, where the assumption of proportional hazards can be justified.

REVIEW QUESTIONS

1. In what circumstances might survival analysis tools be recommended rather than other, potentially simpler, analytical methods?
2. What are the two main tools used in survival analysis and how do they differ?
3. Think of some study or research questions where you might want to use survival analysis methods.

SUGGESTED FURTHER READING

Bull K, Spiegelhalter DJ. Tutorial in biostatistics: survival analysis in observational studies. Statistics in Medicine. 1997:16:1041–74.
Kirkwood BR, Sterne JAC. Essential medical statistics, 2nd ed. Carlton: Blackwell Science, 2006, pp. 272–94.
Pocock SJ, Clayton TC, Altman DG. Survival plots of time-to-event outcomes in clinical trials: good practice and pitfalls. Lancet. 2002;359:1686–9.

REFERENCES

1. Pocock SJ, Clayton TC, Altman DG. Survival plots of time-to-event outcomes in clinical trials: good practice and pitfalls. Lancet. 2002;359:1686–9.
2. Bull K, Spiegelhalter DJ. Tutorial in biostatistics: survival analysis in observational studies. Statistics in Medicine. 1997:16:1041–74.
3. Kirkwood BR, Sterne JAC. Essential medical statistics, 2nd ed. Carlton: Blackwell Science, 2006, pp. 272–94.

Explaining the Why (Qualitative)

This section describes some of the more common qualitative methods of enquiry. It is not intended as a comprehensive summary of all the approaches that may be employed to analyse non-numerical data, but rather covers methods that may be of relevance to paramedicine.

Qualitative research helps to explore a phenomenon of interest, investigate a person's lived experiences or describe attitudes, beliefs and values held by individuals or group members.

Data collection may involve focus groups or interviews that aim to understand the perceptions and experiences of individuals that are the focus of the research question. For example, a research question such as 'What are the experiences of children who are seen by a paramedic after sustaining an injury?' seeks to explore the child's experience, their understanding and meanings associated with this encounter. This type of question cannot be adequately answered by a retrospective analysis of patient care records. Instead, the researcher will need to design a study that aims to capture the child's experience as well as the meanings or understandings associated with this interaction.

Qualitative research has been the subject of criticism for lack of rigour in the use of established methods of enquiry and poor justification for the use of the reported method. Studies that lack a clear description of the approach used to analysing, interpreting and reporting data can raise questions about the validity and reliability of the data. Whereas a research question that asks about measurable differences between groups requires specific research methods such as a t-test or ANOVA, there are several methods that may be suitable to explore the child's experience of their interactions with paramedics. This chapter provides examples of methods that may be suitable for collecting and analysing qualitative data. However, it is important that the method be fit for purpose and the process for collecting, analysing and interpreting the data must be rigorous and true to the method.

Many important aspects of paramedicine can be answered using qualitative research, in particular research that aims to understand the patient's experiences, so that the results can inform safe and effective patient-centred care.

35

Phenomenology

William J Leggio

LEARNING OUTCOMES

1. Define phenomenology qualitative research
2. Describe research questions appropriate for phenomenological inquiry
3. Discuss steps in conducting phenomenology qualitative research

INTRODUCTION

Phenomenology is an approach of qualitative research and is a methodology focused on understanding a specific phenomenon. Phenomenological research is a form of narrative research to understand the essence of an experience, or the phenomenon.[1] A phenomenological study typically collects qualitative data from individuals or focus groups. Data collected serves as a narrative to describe experiences in support of understanding a common meaning of the phenomenon.[1] Data is then analysed, typically performing a thematic analysis, to develop a description of the phenomenon for all the individuals.[1]

Phenomenological research can be a standalone qualitative research project or it can be part of a mixed methods inquiry. For example, phenomenology may be used as phase 2 of an explanatory sequential mixed methods design to have participants help explain quantitative findings.[2] A phenomenological approach may be first used during an exploratory sequential mixed methods design to aid in constructing a new quantitative tool by providing construct validity from the qualitative data.[2]

TRANSCENDENTAL PHENOMENOLOGY, HERMENEUTICAL PHENOMENOLOGY AND BRACKETING

Transcendental phenomenology is best described as collecting data then synthesising significant statements into common themes, whereas hermeneutical phenomenology closely analyses the phenomenon and reflects on essential themes as an interpretation of the meaning of the phenomenon.[1] Though similar, the use of data and themes either describes a phenomenon (transcendental) or tries to explain the phenomenon (hermeneutical). Bracketing can be included as part of the process for both approaches. Bracketing is when the researcher(s) identifies and develops an awareness of their own experiences and biases related to the phenomenon to either be bracketed out during data synthesis (transcendental) or used as part of interpretation of data (hermeneutical).

GENERAL PROCESSES FOR CONDUCTING PHENOMENOLOGICAL METHODOLOGY

Before Data Collection

As with any research project, it is important to have a clear and focused question. If the research question is about an experience, then the use of phenomenology should be considered. For example, what have been the experiences of paramedics from diverse cultural backgrounds in the emergency medical services (EMS) profession? If chosen, then begin defining the phenomenon and structure for the study. This can be determined by reviewing phenomenological methodology, identifying the need to understand the shared experience including a review of related literature, and reading similar qualitative studies, if available.

Construct a Research Protocol and Data Collection Tool

The use of open-ended questions typically allows for participants to share their own narrative and words in describing the why, how or what of the experience.[1] Writing open-ended questions that are balanced and keep interviews manageable can be a daunting task, but it can be made easier by reading related literature and considering your own experiences as identified through bracketing. Asking a peer(s) and content expert(s) not participating in the study to review originally written open-ended questions is encouraged. After this, it is advisable to pilot the tool and make any final edits before actual data collection. It is important to consider early how data and findings will be validated when designing a phenomenological study, which includes the research protocol and data collection tool(s).

Data Collection

Collecting data during a phenomenological study can be focused on the participant's narrative of the phenomenon. This often means an interview with consent to audio record the session. Audio recording for transcription is encouraged as opposed to note taking during the interview as the act of note taking can distract participants and diminish the researcher's ability to listen actively and be present. Other forms of data may be collected such as observations and journals.[1,2]

There is no specific number of interviews or participants required to collect data from for a phenomenological study. It is generally thought 5 to 25 participants that experienced the phenomenon is an appropriate range.[1] There are many factors that influence an exact number for any phenomenology study, including the actual number of individuals that experienced a phenomenon.

Drawing on the principles of qualitative methodologies, reaching saturation is a dynamic guide to help determine the number of study participants. Saturation is reached when no new data or information is being collected from participants.[1,2] The concept of reaching saturation can be subjective as it likely does not fully exclude the possibility of discovering new information from additional participants. However, reaching saturation remains a pragmatic approach to determining when to end data collection to perform a thematic analysis.

Reporting the Phenomenon

There are many ways to organise and prepare phenomenological data. Themes of significant statements or observations can be organised manually or with the use of software. Performing a review for significance in data is followed by developing textual and structural descriptions. Textual and structural statements should develop descriptions of the phenomenon and provide context, setting(s) and commonality or variance to the individual experiences.[1] An understanding of the essence of the phenomenon should emerge from the textual and structural statements.[1]

Validating Data and Reporting

Phenomenology and other forms of qualitative research can be scrutinised by concerns for the validity of the results.[3] As previously mentioned, considering early on how data and results will be validated should be considered early in the study design. Establishing creditability and validity can start with bracketing and including reviewers not involved in the project during the study design.[3]

There are multiple ways to determine validity in qualitative research, and having multiple approaches is suggested.[2,3] Three techniques for determining validity to consider with phenomenology are member checking, triangulation and use of an auditor.

Member checking is involving study participants in validating data and has been described as the most crucial approach in establishing creditability and validity.[3] There are many ways to facilitate the process, but the intent is to provide participants data and themes. Participants are asked if the reporting makes sense, is sufficient and overall account is accurate.

Triangulation is a process in confirming or disconfirming data. Using findings from a similar study, facts from external authoritative sources and the content of related theories are examples of confirming or disconfirming data.[3]

The use of an auditor is similar to peer review as part of the study design. An auditor is essentially presented with the entire study and documentation and asked to review whether both the process and product are appropriate and justified.[3]

EXAMPLES

Two published phenomenological studies are shared as examples. The first example is from rural western Sweden and researched how ambulance personnel prepare themselves for everyday assignments.[4] In the study, a researcher embedded themselves with ambulance team members to observe prehospital care situations and the personnel's day-to-day lives. Field notes were taken to document observations made during 25 prehospital care situations in addition to interviews with ambulance personnel before and after each patient encounter. All research data was coded to provide a general structure of the phenomenon to form three themes.[4] Strengths of the study include application of reflective lifeworld research, the steps taken to not influence patient encounters and general findings to support the importance of the relationship of patient assessment to patient outcomes.[4] Weaknesses of the study were described within the limitations, which included data being collected from crews at a single station.[4]

The second example sought to better understand the experiences of homeless shelter users as EMS patients.[5] In the study, data was obtained from structured interviews with homeless shelter users that were once EMS patients.[5] Interviews were conducted by undergraduate EMS students with the audio recorded and transcribed for phenomenological thematic analysis.[5] Strengths of this study included the use of significant quotes in the manuscript to support themes and discussing study findings that supported related literature.[5] Weaknesses and limitations of the study included the inability to conduct member checking of the data as well as use of a convenient sample of individuals seeking services from a single homeless shelter that were identified by shelter staff as once being an EMS patient.[5]

Both examples received approval from an institutional review board and were published in notable journals. This serves as evidence to the willingness of journals to publish phenomenological research. Both examples added value to the paramedicine body of knowledge through increased understanding of phenomena that are difficult to quantify. Neither study attempted to overstate results and appropriately recognised limitations of the reporting in addition to identifying areas for future research.

CONCLUSION

Research using discrete data such as numerical values (e.g. dispatch times or vital signs) or binary categorical forms (e.g. performed/not performed or successful/not successful) are important to the paramedicine profession. However, statistics without a narrative can just be numbers providing limited meaning. There is much more to the profession than just numbers. There are humans with narratives rich in experience and non-quantifiable perspectives. As such, phenomenology provides a research approach using narratives placed in context with an effort to increase understanding of a shared phenomenon.

REVIEW QUESTIONS

1. In your own words, describe phenomenological research.
2. How would you frame a phenomenological research question based on an experience you had and feel paramedicine needs to better understand?
3. How would you approach conducting a phenomenological inquiry based on your identified experience?

SUGGESTED FURTHER READING

Creswell JW, Poth CN. Qualitative inquiry & research design: choosing among five approaches. 4th ed. Los Angeles: SAGE; 2018.

REFERENCES

1. Creswell JW, Poth CN. Qualitative inquiry & research design: choosing among five approaches. 4th ed. Los Angeles: SAGE; 2018.
2. Creswell JW, Creswell JD. Research design: qualitative, quantitative and mixed-methods approaches. 5th ed. Los Angeles: SAGE; 2018.
3. Creswell JW, Miller DL. Determining validity in qualitative inquiry. Theory and Practice. 2000 Aug;39(3):124–30.
4. Sundström BW, Dahlberg K. Being prepared for the unprepared: a phenomenology field study of Swedish prehospital care. Journal of Emergency Nursing. 2012 Nov;38(6):571–7.
5. Leggio WJ, Giguere A, Sininger C, Zlotnicki N, Walker S, Miller MG. Homeless shelter users and their experiences as EMS patients: a qualitative study. Prehospital Emergency Care. 2020 Mar 3;24(2):214–9.

36

Action Research Methodology for Out-of-Hospital Care Researchers

Sam Willis

LEARNING OUTCOMES

1. Define action research
2. Identify the stages of the action research cycle
3. Recognise how to apply action research in the out-of-hospital setting

INTRODUCTION

Action research is commonly used in the social sciences as a methodology for improving clinical practice. It combines experiential learning, observation and reflection, which can lead to tangible changes in clinical practice. While there are no universally accepted definitions of action research, current definitions centre around its purpose in the research world.[1] For example, Reason and Bradbury identify action research as a study design that informs and influences practice, making it a preferable choice for paramedics considering undertaking research to improve their clinical practice or who are enrolled into a research degree.[2]

Action research is also known as participatory action research (PAR), community-based study, cooperative inquiry and action science and there are many different types including diagnostic action research, participant action research, empirical action research and experimental action research.[1,3]

THE ACTION RESEARCH CYCLE

The action research process is cyclical and consists of the following four stages: planning, action, observation and reflection.

Planning

Planning involves thinking about all the possible options for improving practice. It often includes talking with others or designing a process of investigation.

Action

When taking action, this involves considering what has been learned about the situation, having undertaken a reflection or spoken with others, and executing a plan. In the context of research, it refers to undertaking data collection.

Observation

Observation may have been something that was observed by others, observed directly by the researcher or clinician, or might even be a situation that the researcher has experienced first-hand.

Reflection

Reflection as part of action research should be a detailed and structured process, using a framework that will guide a deeper understanding of the situation, as opposed to a quick chat with a friend.

ADVANTAGES AND DISADVANTAGES

Action research, like all other methods, has advantages and disadvantages. Advantages include the aims of action research being a process orientated to learning and one which includes others, as opposed to a single researcher.[2] Such a view aligns to social constructivist theories of knowledge formation as a social experience, bringing all those benefits associated with social constructionism.[4] Such an approach allows real-world issues to be discussed, explored and resolved, as opposed to investigating abstract ideas that do not help us to perform better in our world.

In contrast, action research requires the commitment of time and effort for planning and implementation,[5] including maintaining collaborative networks, which can be perceived as a time-consuming process when compared to other techniques. Action research also relies on others, meaning if group members stop attending, the process is jeopardised.

APPLYING THE CYCLE IN PRACTICE

When applying action research to a project or process of improvement, it is commonplace to use the cycles more than once during a study or process of improvement, as will be discussed. Also worth noting is that some authors choose to implement these stages in a different sequence to that just described, in order to suit their needs. To highlight our point, we will use cycles of research (see Fig 36.1) which starts at the observation stage as follows: observe, reflect, plan and act.[6] O'Leary's cycles of research are used to structure the following examples.

EXAMPLE 1

Case Study

Gian is a paramedic manager who has been working for a large ambulance service for many years. Recently the service changed from a paper-based patient care record (PCR) system to a completely new, electronic system, replacing handwritten PCRs with electronic PCRs (ePCR) using an iPad.

Cycle 1

Shortly after launching the new system, Gian **observed** that his staff were spending longer on scene and spending more time at hospital. When he **reflected** on this using the Gibbs (1988) reflective model,[7] he concluded that he wouldn't ignore it, hoping that it resolved itself. Instead he was proactive and decided that he would speak with staff about their experiences. As he did so, staff reported the new electronic PCRs as problematic, and each staff member highlighted a slightly different concern.

Gian decided to explore this further to help resolve the situation and started by **planning** a short five-question paper-based survey to collect data more formally. Following approval from his employer and the ambulance service ethics department, he took **action** and distributed the survey to the staff in his area. When he analysed the results, they showed that, on average staff were having to access five different screens just to input a set of patient vital signs. He also found that the overall layout was not easy to navigate, which not only delayed paramedics on scene and

at hospital, but also caused frustration and lack of satisfaction among the staff.

Cycle 2

Having immersed himself in the data, **observing** the key challenges facing paramedics, he **reflected** on the larger situation, including the potential downfalls of not resolving the matter. He also reflected in detail on all his options for taking the issue further. Having reflected on his options, Gian **planned** to contact the executive management team to show them the evidence, highlighting how the situation affected ambulance response times, ambulance availability, hospital ramping, patient safety and staff satisfaction. His next steps were to take **action** by arranging a meeting with the executive leadership team, which he did the following week.

As a result of presenting his case, the executive team started by distributing Gian's survey to the entire service. The data overwhelmingly supported the data supplied by the staff in Gian's local area, and as a result, the necessary changes were made to the ePCR. This had the effect of reducing delays on scene and at hospital, and increasing staff satisfaction.

Example 2
Case Study

Sarah is a newly qualified paramedic, studying for an honours degree. This requires the planning and design of a detailed research project and she has chosen to use an action research methodology as she has read of its ability to create change.

Cycle 1

Since qualifying and working as a paramedic, she **observed** how not all student paramedics get a comparable experience from their mentors during work-integrated learning (WIL). When **reflecting** on this using the cycle of Willis, she remembered situations that affected her during her studies.[7] She also undertook a literature review that identified how student paramedics struggle to fit in when they arrive for WIL, which affects their overall confidence and ability to achieve many of their university learner outcomes. When **planning** her study, she decided to use interviews for data collection (**acting**) and from the interview data found that students not only have a deep desire to fit in on station, but that they fear being made to look silly in front of their peers by their mentors and other paramedics. As a result, they sit quietly during crucial interactions and exclude themselves from any situation that might humiliate them. As Sarah was undertaking the research for a qualification, her role was to demonstrate an ability to design a research study, execute data collection and analyse and present the data. Therefore, she did not take any further action to resolve the situation, but instead used action research as a methodology and face-to-face interviews as a research method to explore student experiences of WIL.

CONCLUSION

Action research is a process of planning, action, observation and reflection. It has the powerful combined effect of leading to a deeper understanding of a situation and behaviour change. Action research is a suitable methodology for clinical paramedics, educators, students and clinical leaders as a means for changing their practices, solving complex, situated problems and in the context of student paramedics, for use during their education that allows them to explore real-world challenges.

REVIEW QUESTIONS

1. What are the four stages of the action research cycle?
2. O'Leary's cycle of research in Figure 36.1 starts with observation instead of planning. What are some of the advantages of this?
3. Think about your own practice and maybe brainstorm the areas that you feel require exploration. From your brainstorm select one area and describe how the stages of action research might be used to explore and resolve such a matter.

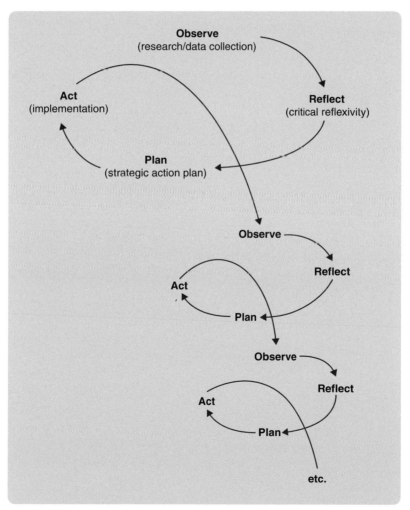

Figure 36.1 O'Leary's cycles of research. (Source: O'Leary Z. The essential guide to doing research. London: SAGE Publications; 2004.)

SUGGESTED FURTHER READING

McNiff J, Whitehead J. All you need to know about action research. London: SAGE Publications, 2011.

REFERENCES

1. Koshy E, Koshy V, Waterman H. Action research in healthcare. London: SAGE Publications, 2011.
2. Reason P, Bradbury H. The SAGE handbook of action research: participative inquiry and practice. 2nd ed. London: SAGE Publications; 2008.
3. Adelman C. Kurt Lewin and the origins of action research. Educational Action Research. 1993;1(1):7–24.
4. Crotty M. The foundations of social research: meaning and perspective in the research process. Sydney: Allen and Unwin; 1998.
5. Hampshire AJ. What is action research and can it promote change in primary care? Journal of Evaluation in Clinical Practice. International Journal of Public Health Policy and Health Services Research. 2008;6(4):337–343.
6. O'Leary Z. The essential guide to doing research. London: SAGE Publications; 2004.
7. Gibbs G (1988). Learning by doing: a guide to teaching and learning methods. Further Education Unit. India: Oxford Polytechnic.

37

Case Study

Ibrahim Althagafi, Lindsay Smith, Dale Edwards and Douglas Paton

LEARNING OUTCOMES

1. Understand how case study research is relevant to the profession of paramedicine
2. Describe three types of case studies (descriptive, exploratory and explanatory)
3. Identify the types and sources of data utilised in case study research
4. Discuss the four elements used to define the case in a case study
5. Be aware of the strengths and weaknesses of case study research in paramedicine

DEFINITION

Case study research is an intensive analysis of an event, unit or phenomenon of interest and its relationships in a naturalistic context that constitute a defined interacting system at the specified point of time through multiple sources of data.

INTRODUCTION

The scope and complexity of paramedicine are rapidly evolving and the paramedic's professional identity is expanding. Understanding such changes and the opportunities brought forward requires a holistic and naturalistic approach. Case study research can offer an appropriate strategy for understanding contemporary phenomenon within a real-life context leading to an in-depth understanding.[1] Often the researcher has little control over the phenomenon and context.[2] In this way, case studies are different to experiments.

Case study research has a long history whose contemporary focus is derived from qualitative research methods across multiple disciplines, including anthropology, history, psychology and sociology to evolve into the research method it is today.[3,4] Case study research continues to evolve from a qualitative research method to include mixed methods case studies.[5]

WHAT ARE THE MAJOR VARIATIONS OF CASE STUDIES?

There are distinctive types of case studies that differ according to their aims and the types of research questions that they ask. These are descriptive, exploratory and explanatory. Yin states that, although overlaps between them exist, they differ according to three main conditions:[2]

1. the type of research question posed
2. the control the researcher has over the actual behavioural events
3. whether the focus is on contemporary versus entirely historical events.

Descriptive case studies focus on 'what' and 'how' research questions to illustrate the operation of an identified general principle.[2,6] Grimes and Schulz consider descriptive case studies to represent a first line of scientific inquiry to understand a phenomenon within healthcare.[7]

Exploratory case studies explore phenomena where there is no clear research question at the beginning of the study.[6] A theoretical proposition (or propositions) based on the prior known evidence is used to guide data collection and analysis to enable theorising and inferences to be drawn.[8]

Explanatory case studies typically focus on the 'why' of a situation.[2] They may utilise multi-case study or a mixed methods methodology and aim to understand the interacting processes and relationships of the case, often over time, and why they result in the impact/outcome observed.[9,10]

DATA INCLUDED IN CASE STUDY RESEARCH

Decisions on the type of data included in the case study, qualitative data or a mix of qualitative and quantitative data, as well as the amount and priority of each, depend on the focus of the case study and the availability of pertinent data. Care in data collection is required to ensure the data accurately engages with the focus of the case study. It can sometimes be difficult to collect data specific to the focus, especially valid quantitative data; hence, many great case studies are qualitative studies. Despite the aforementioned difficulty with quantitative data, mixed methods case studies where both forms of data enhance understanding in health are emerging (see Smith and colleagues for an example).[11]

Qualitative case studies examine multiple sources of qualitative data and may involve scant quantitative data such as demographic details. Mixed-methods case studies incorporate the collection, analysis and integration of both qualitative and quantitative data and other mixed methods research techniques.[5,12] Furthermore, case studies may examine a single case or multiple cases. A single case study facilitates gaining an understanding of 'what' and 'how' something happens. On the other hand, the multiple case study may be useful for cross-analysis and comparison between two cases exploring 'why', replicating and testing theory generated from a single case study.[13,14]

STEPS REQUIRED TO CONDUCT YOUR OWN CASE STUDY RESEARCH

Two steps are necessary to commence a case study research project. First, correctly define the case, its context and background. This step involves a process known as 'bounding the case'.[2] To define the case you must identify the:
- focus of the case study—specifically articulate the event, incident, service phenomenon or phenomena of interest
- relationships connecting with the identified focus
- naturalistic context
- point or points of time to be included.

Together these four elements constitute a defined interacting system at the specified point of time.

The second step in case study research is identifying the types and sources of data available for collection. Types of data may include interviews, review of records, government reports, observations and survey data.

Cases and case notes are integral to paramedicine and can be a source of data in a case study. However, for a project to be considered case study research, theoretical consideration on the defined case and the sources of data

is required; for example, analysis of how the data relates to known theories and/or models in the literature.[8]

STRENGTHS AND WEAKNESSES OF CASE STUDY RESEARCH IN PARAMEDICINE

Case studies allow researchers to examine phenomena that are poorly understood and lack the available data required to facilitate understanding.[15] Case studies offer a high level of detail, richness, completeness and depth and can capture the complexities in the real-life, atypical, threatening and dynamic settings in which paramedics work, making them well suited to paramedicine research practice.[3]

Case study research has limitations emerging from the aim and scope of the study undertaken and difficulty collecting data specific to the focus of the case study. Results may be most pertinent only to the specified local context at the point of time; however, transferability may be appropriate in limited circumstances. Yet multiple case study analyses that test the proposed theory may move closer towards generalisability and causality or more commonly, justify larger higher level studies.[13]

EXAMPLES

While case study has existed in some form throughout the history of paramedicine, there are some noteworthy examples.
- Ford-Jones and Daly explored response of existing paramedic services in Ontario, Canada to an expanding area of mental health-related calls using a case study approach. Three comparative cases, interview's with participants outside the three cases and regional documents were explored.[16]
- Stirling, O'Meara, Pedler, Tourle and Walker used a case study to explore how community engagement by paramedics in an expanded scope role contributes to both primary healthcare and improved emergency response capacity in rural communities. These authors used a multiple case study design, examining four rural ambulance services in Australia.[17]
- Huang, Ma, Sabljak, and Puhala explored the development of community paramedicine (CP) programs in Pennsylvania USA. Their case study used structured interviews from three types of CP programmes: a health system, an ambulance service and an emergency medical service.[18]

CONCLUSION

Case studies are a useful way to explore phenomena in health sciences, as well as other fields. In particular, case studies are useful to explore contemporary issues and unexplained phenomena. Case studies employ a variety of research methods and methodological designs, which include qualitative and mixed methods designs.

REVIEW QUESTIONS

1. When bounding the case in a case study research proposal what four elements are necessary? Use an example from paramedicine to illustrate each element of a proposed (or hypothetical) case study.
2. When reading a case study report, what are the indications of a strong case study and what are the areas of potential weakness to be aware of when considering its transferability to your own practice?

REFERENCES

1. Mills AJ, Durepos G, Wiebe E. Introduction to encyclopaedia of case study research. In: Mills AJ, Durepos G, Wiebe E, editors. Encyclopedia of case study research. Vol. 1. SAGE Publications; 2010, pp. xxxi–xxxiv.
2. Yin RK. Case study research and applications: design and methods. 6th ed. SAGE Publications; 2018.
3. Flyvbjerb B. Case study. In: Norman K. Denzin YSL, editors. The SAGE handbook of qualitative research. 4th ed. SAGE Publications; 2011, pp. 301–16.
4. Harrison H, Birks M, Franklin R, Mills J, editors. Case study research: foundations and methodological orientations. Forum Qualitative Sozialforschung/Forum: Qualitative Social Research; 2017.
5. Plano Clark VL, Ivankova NV. Mixed methods research: a guide to the field. SAGE Publications; 2015.
6. Baxter P, Jack S. Qualitative case study methodology: study design and implementation for novice researchers. The Qualitative Report. 2008;13(4):544–59.
7. Grimes DA, Schulz KF. Descriptive studies: what they can and cannot do. The Lancet. 2002;359(9301):145–9.
8. Mitchell JC. Case and situational analysis. In: Gomm R, Hammersley M, Foster P, editors. Case study method: key issues, key texts. London: SAGE; 2000, pp. 165–86.
9. Gomm R, Hammersley M, Foster P. Case study and generalisation. In: Gomm R, Hammersley M, Foster P, editors. Case study method: key issues, key texts. London: SAGE; 2000, pp. 98–116.
10. Shankardass K, Renahy E, Muntaner C, O'Campo P. Strengthening the implementation of Health in All Policies: a methodology for realist explanatory case studies. Health Policy and Planning. 2015;30(4):462–73.
11. Smith L, Webber R, DeFrain J. Spiritual wellbeing and its relationship to resilience in young people: a mixed methods case study. SAGE Open. 2013;3(2):2158244013485582.
12. Guetterman TC, Fetters MD. Two methodological approaches to the integration of mixed methods and case study designs: a systematic review. American Behavioral Scientist. 2018;62(7):900–18.
13. Stake RE. Multiple case study analysis: Guilford Press; 2006.
14. Ridder H-G. The theory contribution of case study research designs. Business Research. 2017;10(2):281–305.
15. Shaban RZ, Considine J, Fry M, Curtis K. Case study and case-based research in emergency nursing and care: theoretical foundations and practical application in paramedic prehospital clinical judgment and decision-making of patients with mental illness. Australasian Emergency Nursing Journal. 2017;20(1):17–24.
16. Ford-Jones PC, Daly T. Filling the gap: mental health and psychosocial paramedicine programming in Ontario, Canada. Health & Social Care in the Community. 2020.
17. Stirling CM, O'Meara P, Pedler D, Tourle V, Walker J. Engaging rural communities in health care through a paramedic expanded scope of practice. Rural and Remote Health. 2007;7(4):1.
18. Huang Y-H, Ma L, Sabljak LA, Puhala ZA. Development of sustainable community paramedicine programmes: a case study in Pennsylvania. Emergency Medicine Journal. 2018;35(6):372–8.

38

Ethnography: A Process and Product

Louise Reynolds

LEARNING OUTCOMES

1. Define ethnography
2. Appraise the strengths and weaknesses of ethnography in relation to paramedicine research
3. Describe the various ethnographic data collection methods
4. Evaluate the contribution of ethnography to paramedicine research

DEFINITIONS

- Ethnography: A research approach that describes the culture of a particular group.
- Participant observation: A method for data collection whereby the researcher spends time, unobtrusively, observing participant's behaviour, actions and interactions so that they can understand and make sense of the constructed meanings of their environment and everyday life.[1]
- Interview: A method for data collection which seeks to gain an understanding of the participant's assumptions and social reality.[2]
- Field notes: A method for data collection which records a researcher's observations and or participation in the field.[3]
- Autoethnography: A process and product of a cultural description in which the researcher is the focus of the data collection method.
- Critical ethnography: A process and product of a cultural description which examines the relationship of culture and power relationships.[4]
- Interpretative ethnography: The generation of descriptions by way of 'walking in the shoes' of participants in order to gain a sense of the practices that define the workplace culture.[4-6]
- Feminist ethnography: A cultural description through the lens of feminist theory.[1]

INTRODUCTION

Imagine a researcher observing the care of birthing mothers in a community with many cultural differences that have not been previously described. If they are invited to be an observer, the researcher may wish to record interactions between the mother and carers during and following the birth of a child. They may also record their observations of behaviours, cultural norms, social support, the influence of spiritual beliefs and access to healthcare in the community to develop a comprehensive understanding of the significance of their observations.

The research activity of observation, participation, interview and fieldnotes is classic ethnography. Ethnography is both a process and product which documents the culture of a particular group.[6] This means that researchers use ethnography as research design and their final research report is called an ethnography.

STRENGTHS AND WEAKNESSES OF THIS DESIGN

The strength of this design is being able to study people and their behaviours in their natural environment, which means that the account is authentic and contextual.[7] This is called a 'thick description' which means that the researcher is able to immerse themselves in the context of the culture they are describing in detail.[8] This kind of detail means that the ethnographer has the ability to draw from multiple sources and types of data.

The risk or challenge for ethnographers is 'going or being native'; that is, being immersed in the field and not being able to gain the perspective needed.[9] Some strategies to help the researcher in gaining perspective include keeping a reflective journal and collaborating with other critical friends and readers during data analysis.

Like other qualitative methodologies, there are a number of strategies that can be used to ensure rigour.[10,11] This means that ethnographers need to ensure that they are collecting data that is 'trustworthy' meaning it is creditable, transferable, dependable and able to be confirmed.[10,11] This can be achieved by a range of strategies such as spending enough time in data collection, documenting decisions during data collection, considering the application of the findings and having a range of voices represented.[10,11]

Generally, qualitative research is criticised for validity and reliability due to its subjective nature and small sample size.[11] These claims have been addressed elsewhere in the literature which means that ethnographers as qualitative researchers should focus on a rigorous design.[12]

STEPS REQUIRED TO CONDUCT YOUR OWN STUDY OF THIS DESIGN

Starting with your question, which would focus on the 'what' of a particular group which relates to the cultural elements of values, beliefs, symbols and rituals.[13] This means that the process and production of the cultural description is central to the intended outcome.

In order to generate a 'thick description', an ethnography collects data using a variety of methods. These include participant observation, interviews, field notes and documents.[1,7,14]

Ethnographic interviews seek to describe the context and construction of a participant's understanding of their environment.[2] Interview format will depend on the ethnographer's intention for depth and quality of information.[15] Interviews in this case intend to be a rich source of 'sense making' of culture when participants use the specific language, convey beliefs and values and describe symbolic rituals or practices.[16]

There are two methods of participant observation: participation and or observation.[1] As a data collection method, it is intended to be unobtrusive by spending time in the 'field' to describe the everyday experiences. It enables the ethnographer to understand the complex social setting as they move from being the complete participant, participant-observer and complete observer.[17] The record of participant observation is recorded as a field note.[3]

Once the data has been collected, it is aggregated and thematically analysed.[15] Ethnographic data analysis is a continual, iterative process throughout data collection to ensure that there was a 'feedforward' opportunity to clarify understanding at the next opportunity for data collection.[18] Themes are arranged into a scheme or taxonomy, which are coded categories when looking for similarly grouped ideas.[3,19,20]

There are a number of variations to ethnography: interpretative, critical, feminist and autoethnography.[1,7,14] Each of these variations view the cultural description with a different theoretical lens. This means that, depending on how and what question is being asked regarding the cultural description, the researcher may wish to look further at gender (feminist ethnography), power relationships (critical ethnography) or their own relationship (autoethnography).[7,14]

EXAMPLES OF PARAMEDICINE-FOCUSED ETHNOGRAPHY

Early ethnographies in the United States described the emerging work of paramedics during the 1980s.[21–24] Palmer described ambulance workers as 'trauma junkies' while Mannon and Metz account for the highly ritualised and stressful operational environment.[22,25–27]

Australian ethnographer Reynolds has described the organisational culture in a jurisdictional ambulance service, while Boyle focused their description of ambulance organisational culture on the relationship of emotional work aspect and masculinity.[28,29] Using autoethnography, Furness, Lehmann and Gardner described ambulance work as a reflective account.[30]

In the United Kingdom, McCann and colleagues described the professionalisation in relation to the National Health Service.[31]

As a research process, O'Meara and colleagues used ethnographic observation methods to describe rural Canadian community paramedicine.[32] This allowed the researchers to immerse themselves in the program, both as a process and for the production of the description.

CONCLUSION

Ethnography is a qualitative methodology that is a process and product of a cultural description. For paramedicine research, ethnography has already provided a rich and 'thick description' of the work, workers and workplace.

REVIEW QUESTIONS

1. From your experience in ambulance services, what can you identify as paramedic culture?
2. List the various data collection methods that ethnographers can use to collect data in an ambulance service.

3. What, if any, potential ethical issues are related to data collection when undertaking participant observation?
4. You are considering undertaking a feminist ethnography to describe ambulance culture. What potential issues relating to paramedicine practice might you wish to explore?

SUGGESTED FURTHER READING

Furness SE, Lehmann J, Gardner F. Autoethnographic analysis of the self through an occupational story of a paramedic. Journal of Paramedic Practice. 2016;8(12):589-95.

McCann L, Granter E, Hyde P, Hassard J. Still blue-collar after all these years? An ethnography of the professionalization of emergency ambulance work. Journal of Management Studies. 2013;50(5):750-76. Online. Available: https://doi.org/10.1111/joms.12009.

REFERENCES

1. Grbich C, editor. Qualitative research in health: an introduction. St Leonards: Allen & Unwin; 1998.
2. Hammersely M. Recent radical criticism of interview studies: any implications for the sociology of education? British Journal of Sociology of Education. 2003;24(1):119–26.
3. Emerson RM, Fritz RI, Shaw LL. Writing ethnographic fieldnotes. Chicago: University of Chicago Press; 1995.
4. Angus LB. Research traditions, ideology and critical ethnography. Discourse. 1986;7(1):61–77.
5. Angus LB. Developments in ethnographic research in education: from interpretative to critical ethnography. Journal of Research and Development in Education. 1986;20(1):59–67.
6. Hammersely M, Atkinson P. Ethnography: principles in practice. 2nd ed. London: Routledge; 1995.
7. Green J, Thorogood N. Qualitative methods for health research. 4th ed. Los Angeles: SAGE; 2018.
8. Geertz C. The interpretation of cultures: selected essays. New York, USA: Basic Books, Inc.; 1973.
9. O'Reilly K. Key concepts in ethnography. Los Angeles: SAGE; 2009.
10. Morse J, Barrett M, Mayan M, Olsen K, Spiers J. Verification strategies for establishing reliability and validity in qualitative research. International Journal of Qualitative Methods. 2002;2(1):1–19.
11. Lincoln YS, Guba EG. Naturalistic inquiry. Beverley Hills, CA: Sage Publications; 1985.
12. de Laine M. Ethnography: theory and applications in health research. Sydney, Australia: Maclennan + Petty; 1997.
13. Schein EH. Culture: the missing concept in organization studies. Administrative Science Quarterly. 1996;41(2):229–41.
14. Flick U. An introduction to qualitative research. 4th ed. London: Sage Publications; 2009.
15. Minichiello V, Madison J, Hays T, Parmenter G. Doing qualitative in-depth interviews. In: Minichiello V, Sullivan G, Greenwood K, Axford R, editors. Research methods for nursing and health science. 2nd ed. Frenchs Forest: Pearson Education Australia; 2004, pp. 629–66.
16. Weick K. Making sense of the organization. Malden, USA: Blackwell Publishing; 2001.
17. Agar MH. The professional stranger: an informal introduction to ethnography. New York: Academic Press; 1980.
18. Bogdan RC, Biklen SK. Qualitative research for education. 3rd ed. Boston, Mass: Allyn and Bacon; 1998.
19. Spradley JP. The ethnographic interview. New York, NY: Holt, Rinehart & Winston; 1979.
20. Spradley JP. Participant observation. New York, NY: Holt, Rinehart and Winston; 1980.
21. Palmer CE. 'Trauma junkies' and street work: occupational behavior of paramedics and emergency medical technicians. Urban Life. 1983;12(2):162–83.
22. Metz D. Running hot: structure and stress in ambulance work. Cambridge: Apt Books; 1981.
23. Mannon J. Emergency encounters: EMTs and their work. Port Washington: Kennikat Press; 1981.
24. Douglas D. Occupational and therapeutic contingencies of ambulance services in metropolitan areas [PhD thesis]: University of California; 1969.
25. Palmer CE. 'Trauma junkies' and street work: Occupational behavior of paramedics and emergency medical technicians. Urban Life. 1983;12(2):162–83.
26. Mannon JM. Emergency encounters: EMTs and their work. Port Washington, NY: Kennikat Press; 1981.
27. Mannon JM. Aiming for 'detached concern'—how EMT's and paramedics cope. Emergency Medical Services. 1981;10(6):11–14, 19–20, passim.
28. Reynolds L. Beyond the front line: an interpretative ethnography of an ambulance service University of South Australia; 2008.
29. Boyle M. Love the work, hate the system [PhD thesis]. St Lucia: University of Queensland; 1997.
30. Furness SE, Lehmann J, Gardner F. Autoethnographic analysis of the self through an occupational story of a paramedic. Journal of Paramedic Practice. 2016;8(12):589–95.
31. McCann L, Granter E, Hyde P, Hassard J. Still blue-collar after all these years? An ethnography of the professionalization of emergency ambulance work. Journal of Management Studies. 2013;50(5):750–76.
32. O'Meara P, Stirling C, Ruest M, Martin A. Community paramedicine model of care: an observational, ethnographic case study. BMC Health Services Research. 2016;16(1):39.

39

Grounded Theory: An Interpretation of Social Reality

David Long

LEARNING OUTCOMES

1. Define grounded theory
2. Differentiate the approaches to grounded theory
3. Evaluate the suitability of grounded theory methodology in paramedicine research

DEFINITION

Grounded theory is a research methodology used for the collection and analysis of qualitative data to produce a theory *grounded* in the data.[1,2] Simply put, theory is a set of interrelated statements that explain something about the social phenomena under investigation.[2] Grounded theory is particularly useful to generate a theory where the primary research question asks, 'What is happening or going on here?'

Grounded theory can be argued to be both a 'method' and 'methodology'. A method refers to techniques and procedures for gathering and analysing data whereas methodology refers to a set of principles and ideas that inform the design of a research study.[2,3] For clarity, this chapter subscribes to the Charmazian view of grounded theory being both a method and methodology.[4]

INTRODUCTION

Grounded theory (GT) was first developed in the 1960s and is among the most common qualitative research methodologies utilised in recent times.[5,6] The popularity of GT is likely related to the adaptability of GT methodology in addressing a wide variety of research questions across numerous disciplines. However, GT is particularly well suited to studying *processes*; that is, sequences of events with a clear beginning and end that can be defined over time.[1] For instance, Reay and colleagues utilised GT methodology to develop a theory to explain the process of how paramedics make decisions in the prehospital setting.[7] Ultimately, GT methodology goes far beyond simply generating a descriptive narrative of events. It aims to explore comprehensively *how* and *why* social actions, events, relationships and behaviours occur the way they do.

Unique approaches to GT methodology can be distinguished across the philosophical spectrum from positivist (objective) through to constructivist (subjective) worldviews. Positivist researchers tend to view the social world through a more objective lens in which data collection and analysis is conducted mostly independently of the researcher's influence to render a singular worldview, whereas constructivists argue reality is a *construction* of their own perceptions, perspectives and experiences in which there is no one 'true' social reality. For this reason, it is important that the researcher identify their ontological (the nature of reality[8]) and epistemological (how knowledge is created[9,10]) orientation to data collection and analysis.[11] In this way, the researcher is explicit about their biases and the 'lens' through which the data has been interpreted.

GROUNDED THEORY METHODOLOGY

After identifying the research question or an area of research enquiry suitable for GT methodology, researchers may begin by seeking out sensitising concepts. As GT does not begin with an a priori theory, sensitising concepts provide the researcher with tentative concepts and ideas to guide the research process. For instance, previous studies may provide some insights into a proposed area of research. Those insights may act as a point of departure for determining data collection strategies including the recruitment of participants.

While a variety of data collection strategies can be utilised in GT including observations, journals, policy documents and photographs, purposive sampling of participants for interviews is perhaps the most common strategy for generating data in GT research. Purposive sampling selects participants based on their exposure, background or experience to speak authoritatively about the topic under investigation. Participants are often interviewed as individuals or in focus groups to generate data in the form of interview transcripts. The data is subsequently analysed and distilled through a process of initial coding and focused coding.[1] In essence, coding attributes a short word or phrase that gives analytic meaning to a portion of data in a similar way that a book title tries to capture the essence of its content.[6] A helpful maxim in the coding process is to simply ask oneself, 'What is going on here?'[2]

Coding and analysis continues through an iterative ('back and forth') process whereby data is inductively analysed and reintegrated into subsequent data collection activities, such as participant interviews, to achieve 'theoretical usefulness'.[1] Through this distillation process, constant comparison and theoretical sampling facilitate the consolidation of codes into theoretical categories (themes).

Constant comparison is a technique whereby the researcher attempts to make analytic distinctions between data sets (e.g. two sets of interviews) to find similarities and differences. A deeper understanding of the similarities and differences between participants can lend fresh insights to the research which can be reintegrated throughout the analytic process. Similarly, theoretical sampling contributes to analytic precision by actively seeking out people, events or information to refine the boundaries and properties of the theoretical categories. Theoretical sampling differs from purposive sampling through the application of deductive reasoning in refining the researcher's understanding of the theoretical categories. Data collection continues until no new insights or patterns are discerned, with theory construction being the endpoint of the GT process (Fig 39.1).

EXAMPLES

Kelly is a researcher who is interested in how paramedics transition to become critical care flight paramedics. Kelly selects GT methodology to develop a theoretical model to explain how the process of transition works. She begins by searching the existing literature for sensitising concepts and finds information on how practitioners in paramedicine and other health fields transition to specialist roles. Kelly then recruits key stakeholders who are likely to be knowledgeable of the transition process including current and former flight paramedics, specialist operations educators and helicopter emergency medical service (HEMS) managers. Sensitising concepts provide a starting point in the participant interviews with data generated via transcripts of the interviews. Kelly codes the data after each interview, thereby gaining new theoretical insights in each step of the analytic process. Codes are distilled to focus codes and so forth until the analysis leads to the development of theoretical (conceptual) categories. Finally, theoretical sampling and returning to the literature lends greater analytic precision to the categories and a theory of transition from paramedic to critical care flight paramedic emerges.

STRENGTHS AND WEAKNESSES OF THIS DESIGN

The strength of GT methodology is that it allows researchers to gain a deeper understanding of a social process or phenomena through a rigorous and systematic approach.[12] The end users of the research, such as clinicians, managers, educators and policy makers, can use the new knowledge to inform a wide variety of domains including workforce planning, paramedic education, clinical practice and future research.

In contrast, GT has known limitations such as the transferability or applicability of the findings to other settings. Consequently, qualitative researchers tend not to advocate for the 'generalisation' of findings to other populations or settings. Rather, the transferability of findings is based on the thick descriptions of the research setting and the conceptual understanding of the relationships between categories.

CONCLUSION

Regardless of the researcher's tendencies towards positivist or constructivist worldviews, GT methodology is best regarded as a set of systematic yet flexible and iterative actions in which the coding and analysis of data aims to achieve a deeper understanding of social phenomena. Constructivist researchers tend to interact with the data more dynamically in accepting that they are not neutral observers in the research process. Either way, the endpoint of GT is to produce a theory or comprehensive explanation of social phenomena grounded in the data.

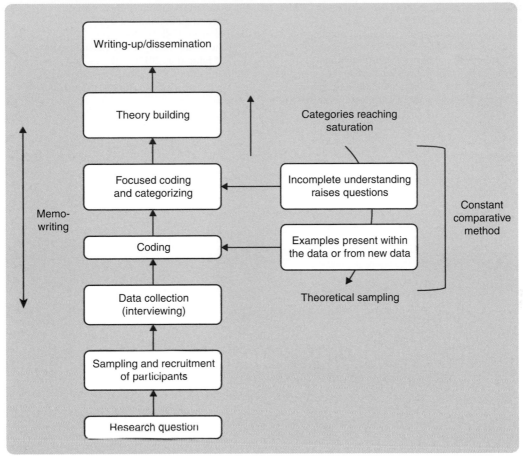

Figure 39.1 A visual representation of grounded theory. (Source: Charmaz K. Constructing grounded theory. 2nd ed. London: SAGE; 2014, p. 18.)

REVIEW QUESTIONS

1. What types of research questions can be answered using grounded theory methodology?
2. What is the difference between purposive sampling and theoretical sampling?
3. How is 'analytic precision' achieved in grounded theory research?

SUGGESTED FURTHER READING

Charmaz K. Constructing grounded theory. 2nd ed. London: SAGE; 2014.
Corbin J, Strauss A. Basics of qualitative research. 4th ed. Thousand Oaks, California: SAGE; 2015.
Saldaña J. The coding manual for qualitative researchers. London: SAGE; 2015.

REFERENCES

1. Charmaz K. Constructing grounded theory. 2nd ed. London: SAGE; 2014.
2. Corbin J, Strauss A. Basics of qualitative research. 4th ed. Thousand Oaks, California: SAGE; 2015.
3. Birks M, Mills J. Grounded theory: a practical guide. Los Angeles: SAGE; 2011.
4. Charmaz K. Special invited paper: continuities, contradictions and critical inquiry in grounded theory. International Journal of Qualitative Methods. 2017;16(1):1–8.
5. Morse J, Stern P, Corbin J, Bowers B, Charmaz K, Clarke A. Developing grounded theory: the second generation: Routledge; 2016.
6. Saldaña J. The coding manual for qualitative researchers. London: SAGE; 2015.
7. Reay G, Rankin J, Smith-MacDonald L, Lazarenko G. Creative adapting in a fluid environment: an explanatory model of

paramedic decision making in the pre-hospital setting. BMC Emergency Medicine. 2018;18(1):1–11.

8. Grix J. Introducing students to the generic terminology of social research. Politics. 2002;22(3):175–86.

9. Scotland J. Exploring the philosophical underpinnings of research: Relating ontology and epistemology to the methodology and methods of the scientific, interpretive and critical research paradigms. English Language Teaching. 2012;5(9):9–16.

10. Urquhart C. Grounded theory for qualitative research: a practical guide. London: SAGE; 2012.

11. Twining P, Heller R, Nussbaum M, Tsai C. Some guidance on conducting and reporting qualitative studies. Computers and Education. 2017;106:1–9.

12. Liamputtong P. Qualitative research methods. 3rd ed. South Melbourne: Oxford University Press; 2009.

40

Data Collection Methods for Qualitative Research

Brendan Shannon

LEARNING OUTCOMES

1. Be able to describe what qualitative data is

2. Justify when you would collect qualitative data and why certain data collection approaches may or may not suit your research methodology

DEFINITIONS

- Qualitative data: Data that describes and characterises a concept; it can be derived from a myriad of sources.
- Coding: 'The process of analysing qualitative data by taking it apart to see what it yields before putting the data back together in a meaningful way.'[1]

INTRODUCTION

To begin with the basics, it's important we cover just what qualitative data is. No doubt you are thinking that the collection of interviews, writing these interviews into text verbatim (transcription) and analysing them (in one of the many methodologies previously described in other chapters) will result in obtaining qualitative data. Ultimately the text you analyse is the qualitative data, right? Well, at a simplistic level you would be correct that this is the 'data' that we analyse in qualitative research.[2] What we learn as we delve a bit deeper is that qualitative research is not constrained to some form of traditional structured interview, even though this is the most popular or traditional source for data in qualitative research. There are many approaches to collecting qualitative data a researcher can employ, all with the same aim of helping us to understand phenomena

of interest or a research topic. The importance of Chapter 6, which discusses developing your research question, is evident here as it will assist in deciding whether a qualitative approach and whether the chosen methodology is appropriate for your aims.

QUALITATIVE DATA COLLECTION APPROACHES

There are many approaches to deciding which types of data can best meet your research aims in a qualitative project. The following are some qualitative data collection approaches to consider.

- *Interviews*: Typically these are one-on-one interviews that can be conducted face to face or facilitated by technology.[3,4] The traditional interview can vary in technique used. They may be structured where only the pre-set questions are asked and in a pre-determined order, or the more fluid semistructured interview style may be used which is characterised by flexibility in question order and questions asked.
- *Focus group interviews*: This is where a group of participants are asked questions and the interviewer (or interviewers) guides the questions and discussion back to

the area of research inquiry as needed. The key difference with focus groups versus one-on-one interviews is that several participants are interviewed concurrently, and the focus is also more on facilitation of a discussion rather than direct interviewing.[5]

- *Observation*: There also options of collecting meaning from other sources outside of interviews including previously constructed recordings on a subject such as online forums or using preexisting pictures or video.[6,7] A fictious example of this may be analysing patient care records written by paramedics to research attitudes towards patients who frequently call for paramedic care.
- *Story completion*: Participants are asked to complete a scenario or story from what they think will happen next or participants may be asked to draw a picture related to the research area or questions.[8]
- *Object elicitation*: Participants are presented some form of stimulus (such as an object) related to the research topic to assist in gaining new insight alongside interviewing. An example used by the authors in this reference saw participants use objects for oral care in intensive care units as a stimulus to discuss perceptions on pain and discomfort associated with those objects.[9]

At the completion of the initial data collection the data from the participant/source is collated and then analysed. This analysis usually begins with some form of categorisation of parts of the sources collected known as 'coding', and there are many ways to go about data analysis to produce codes.[7] The process of coding to be used will be guided by your particular methodology chosen for your research. It is important to realise that there is no prescriptive right or wrong way to go about data analysis, but that it is important to rigorously follow the chosen methodologically. Criticism of qualitative research tends to stem from lack of rigour in following established research methods and reporting of results. Chapters 41 and 43 discusses qualitative data coding and developing themes in more detail.

CONCLUSION

There are many options available to obtain qualitative data. Careful consideration of which approach best suits your needs before beginning data collection is important. Chapter 41 describes qualitative data collection and management and provides an overview of the steps required to collect and manage the data.

REVIEW QUESTION

1. You have decided to collect qualitative data on paramedic perspectives from across Australia on the management of patients suffering from chronic pain. In initial planning, a colleague suggests that focus groups would be a good data collection approach. Considering the nature of the paramedic workforce, do you agree with this approach as being a practical choice?

SUGGESTED FURTHER READINGS

Barrett D, Twycross A. Data collection in qualitative research. Evidence-based Nursing. July 2018;21(3):63–4.

McLellan E, MacQueen KM, Neidig JL. Beyond the qualitative interview: Data preparation and transcription. Field methods. 2003;15(1):63–84.

REFERENCES

1. Creswell JW, Creswell JD. Research design: qualitative, quantitative, and mixed methods approaches: SAGE publications; 2017.
2. Pope C, Ziebland S, Mays N. Analysing qualitative data. BMJ. 2000;320(7227):114–16.
3. Adams E. The joys and challenges of semi-structured interviewing. Community Practitioner. 2010;83(7).
4. Lobe B, Morgan D, Hoffman KA. Qualitative data collection in an era of social distancing. International Journal of Qualitative Methods. 2020;19:1609406920937875.
5. Dilshad RM, Latif MI. Focus group interview as a tool for qualitative research: an analysis. Pakistan Journal of Social Sciences. 2013;33(1).
6. Drabwell L, Eng J, Stevenson F, King M, Osborn D, Pitman A. Perceptions of the use of alcohol and drugs after sudden bereavement by unnatural causes: analysis of online qualitative data. International Journal of Environmental Research and Public Health. 2020;17(3):677.
7. Braun V, Clarke V. Successful qualitative research: a practical guide for beginners. SAGE Publications; 2013.
8. Moller NP, Clarke V, Braun V, Tischner I, Vossler A. Qualitative story completion for counseling psychology research: a creative method to interrogate dominant discourses. Journal of Counseling Psychology. 2021;68(3):286.
9. Dale CM, Carbone S, Gonzalez AL, Nguyen K, Moore J, Rose L. Recall of pain and discomfort during oral procedures experienced by intubated critically ill patients in the intensive care unit: a qualitative elicitation study. Canadian Journal of Pain. 2020;4(3):19–28.

41

Data Management in Qualitative Research

Brendan Shannon

LEARNING OUTCOMES

1. Justify when you would collect qualitative data
2. Understand the process of managing qualitative data at each stage including recruitment, preparation, collecting and storage of data
3. Understand issues that may arise during the data collection process and describe ethical considerations that must be planned for

DEFINITION

- Transcription: The process of writing/typing out audio recordings verbatim.[1]

INTRODUCTION

So you have decided to venture further into the realm of qualitative approach to answer your research question or area of interest. You have likely consulted with supervisors or peers to discover that collecting data in a spreadsheet and then running a quantitative analysis just isn't a suitable method for answering your research question. Just as quantitative research requires certain statistical test(s) and approaches based on the question and data you have collected, the qualitative approach to research is similar.[2] In this chapter we will explore a general approach to qualitative data collection. The fundamental approach to qualitative data management generally includes the steps of recruitment, preparation, collection and then storage of your data. We will explore some useful tips at each stage so your journey into qualitative research can be as smooth as possible.

Having read previous chapters of this book, what you should now realise is that qualitative data can be derived from many different sources and via a myriad of approaches. Despite the variability in the approaches that exist, there are four major steps a researcher goes through to gain sources to enable data to be coded, analysed and reported. Those steps are:

- recruitment
- preparation
- collection
- storage of data.

RECRUITMENT

Recruitment of participants can be very time consuming and, depending on the method of interviewing, it can also be logistically difficult. You need to consider who your potential participants will be and whether you require participants with a range of demographics.[3] Once you have identified the people who may be included, it's time to start advertising.

How Will You Advertise to Recruit?

Commonly, targeted emails or research flyers (electronic and paper based) will be used in student research. You need to consider this process and the steps used carefully. For example, is there a power differential between the advertiser for the study and the participants being asked to enrol? Participants may feel pressure to enrol, for example, if their direct manager is the one the researchers ask to send out the recruitment email.

How Will Participants Indicate Interest and Book in a Time and Place to be Interviewed?

Will you do this all via email and phone calls? Will participants be able to self-register? Will they have options to do this in a location set by you or in a place familiar to them? There are software packages that can assist in organising and booking participant interview appointments that allow participants to choose a time and place from a list you provide in advance.[4] The process for the potential participants should be easy to use as this increases the chances of successful recruitment.

How Will Participants Know What to Do on the Day of the Interview?

It's important to speak to participants prior to the interview where possible. A good approach is to confirm with participants when their booking is first made. It is also good practice to remind participants of the upcoming booking the day before. This helps clear up any last-minute clashes or potential no-shows, saving everyone valuable time and effort.

PREPARATION

You have started recruitment and now it's time to start preparing for your first interview. Preparation for your data collection method is crucial and proper preparation helps to avoid poor-quality data. There are many logistical challenges to plan for regardless of what method you are using to collect data.

Once Your Participants are Recruited, Its Important You Allocate Sufficient Time for the Interview

Do not underestimate the time interviews take. While there is no prescriptive time on how long the interview may take, it really depends on the engagement between yourself and the participant and the richness of the data.[5] As a rough of idea of how long it may take, you need to allow at least 30 minutes to prepare yourself by going over your questions or the stimulus to be used. The interviews themselves can then range anywhere from 10 minutes to a few hours. Therefore, allocating at least 2 or 3 hours for each interview is recommended.

Ensure You have Good-Quality Recording Equipment and a Backup System

This means ensuring that devices are fully charged and have sufficient storage space. For online interviewing, ensure that the participant's microphone enables a level of audio quality for recording and later transcription. Likewise try and be as familiar as possible with the environment you may be undertaking interviews in; this will make you feel more comfortable and confident which will assist in building connection with participants.[6]

Trial Your Questioning Technique as Well as the Questions Themselves

While your questions have likely already been developed and scrutinised by other research team members and supervisors, it is still a good idea to practice. Do this with others either within or external to your research team and ask for feedback. It's amazing what a trial run can show you regarding strengths and weaknesses of your questions, ordering and technique.[5]

Prepare Yourself to be Flexible in Your Approach to Each Participant

Remember, the questions are there to help guide you through gaining a participant's experiences, attitudes, beliefs or understanding of a topic. Each participant will be different and as such you will need to be flexible. Allow the participant to take you on a journey; you are there to guide them back to the path only when needed.

COLLECTION

The time has now come to conduct your first interview. Once you and your participant are ready to start, the first (and most important) issue to consider is making them feel comfortable. In the same way we know in patient–clinician interactions that the more comfortable the patient is, the more trust and the richer the clinical history we will be, the same goes for conducting research interviews.[7]

After introductions, you should first explain the research topic, process and ground rules focusing especially on how confidentiality and anonymity will be maintained. Allow time for the participant to ask any questions and take the time to answer them. The next practical thing is to ensure that information about the research consent forms approved by the overseeing ethics committee have been read, understood and signed. Conducting the research without informed consent is unethical. Check that recording equipment is operating and turned on and you are now ready to start. Remember when facilitating (not leading) your interview that you will need to have flexibility, as mentioned previously. Go where the participant takes you and bring them back on topic or through to the next question only when needed. An experienced facilitator may be willing to attend the interview and provide guidance.

STORAGE OF DATA

After you have recorded your first interview, it's important to ensure that data is stored to a predefined secured storage space in line with your ethics protocol. The recording should be stored on a secure server or cloud service to ensure that you have a backup. Do this as a matter of priority as soon as your participant(s) has left.

You may choose to have your interviews transcribed. Transcription is the process of writing/typing out audio recordings verbatim.[1] You can do this yourself by listening and typing it (time consuming but low cost) or have this done professionally using a company which provides this service (quick and accurate but often costly). Transcription is not always needed and there are emerging practices where audio recordings can be coded directly.[8] If transcription occurs, as with the audio files, ensure you have backup files saved in a secure storage space in accordance with your ethics protocol. Qualitative data analysis software can be used for storing your audio and transcription files and to keep an electronic record of your coding and analysis process, assisting with transparency.[9] A common software package used is NVivo and while you do not need to necessarily use a software program for data analysis, it should at least be considered.

PREDICT ISSUES THAT MAY ARISE

Preparation and planning are essential for collecting your qualitative data. However, there may be some issues that arise. A common issue you may encounter is that some participants don't engage or talk much and others may dominate the discussion if several people are interviewed concurrently; for example, as a focus group.[3] This may be minimised by making participants feel comfortable and using appropriate lead-in or stimulus questions to help generate rich data. If using focus groups, the group dynamics can be a challenge.[10] At times, some participants may effectively collude with each other (consciously or subconsciously) to exclude some participants or inhibit perspectives brought forward. This takes great skill in facilitation to ensure that you collect a broad collection of views on your topic rather than just the dominant ideas of a few. Lastly, participants may also choose to withdraw consent for the interview before, during or after. At all times this must be respected, and you should not coerce participants to remain in the study. Even if you have already collected data participants may still choose to withdraw consent.

CONCLUSION

Qualitative data collection can be complex. Hopefully when using the approach presented and with careful consideration applied at each step, you should feel confident to begin your qualitative data collection.

REVIEW QUESTIONS

1. You have conducted a focus group with six people. Your audio recording was great and there was great discussion on your research topic. You have transcribed the audio recording and are ready to begin coding this focus group data when you are contacted by one of the participants who wishes to withdraw consent from the study.
   a. How should you handle this request?
   b. What should you now do with the focus group data that has been collected?

SUGGESTED FURTHER READING

Braun V, Clarke V. Successful qualitative research: a practical guide for beginners. SAGE Publications; 2013. (specifically Chapters 4, 5 and 6)

Sutton J, Austin Z. Qualitative research: data collection, analysis and management. The Canadian Journal of Hospital Pharmacy. 2015;68(3):226.

REFERENCES

1. McLellan E, MacQueen KM, Neidig JL. Beyond the qualitative interview: data preparation and transcription. Field Methods. 2003;15(1):63–84.
2. Watson R. Quantitative research. Nursing Standard (2014+). 2015;29(31):44.
3. Braun V, Clarke V. Successful qualitative research: a practical guide for beginners. SAGE Publications; 2013.
4. Alexander HS. Cut out calendaring frustration with Calendly. 2020. Online. Available: https://calendly.com/.
5. Frankel R, Devers K. Study design in qualitative research—1: Developing questions and assessing resource needs. Education for Health. 2000;13(2):251–61.
6. Donalek JG. The interview in qualitative research. Urologic Nursing. 2005;25(2):124–5.
7. Adams E. The joys and challenges of semi-structured interviewing. Community Practitioner. 2010;83(7).
8. Evers JC. From the past into the future. How technological developments change our ways of data collection, transcription and analysis. Paper presented at the Forum Qualitative Sozialforschung/Forum: Qualitative Social Research; 2011.
9. Giesen L, Roeser A. Structuring a team-based approach to coding qualitative data. International Journal of Qualitative Methods. 2020;19:1609406920968700.
10. Morrison-Beedy D, Côté-Arsenault D, Feinstein NF. Maximizing results with focus groups: Moderator and analysis issues. Applied Nursing Research. 2001;14(1), 48–53.

Types of Qualitative Data

Belinda Flanagan

INTRODUCTION

Qualitative data is information collected that describes qualities and characteristics that are non-numerical. There are generally two ways that qualitative data are used, and this normally depends on the question being asked by the researcher. Qualitative descriptive research aims to systematically describe a population. It can answer the 'what', 'where' and 'how' questions through observation but not necessarily the 'why'. Often, the phrase 'descriptive' is used in quantitative terms; however, it can also be used in qualitative research for descriptive purposes.[1] The data may be collected qualitatively, but it is often analysed quantitatively, using frequencies, percentages, averages or other statistical analyses to determine relationships.[2] Qualitative research, however, is more holistic and often involves data from various sources to gain a different understanding of individual participants, including their opinions, perspectives and attitudes.[2] This type of qualitative data describes the 'why'. It may be used to explore people or group's concepts or views, real-life context and sensitive topics where flexibility is required to avoid causing distress.[3]

EXAMPLES OF QUALITATIVE DATA COLLECTION METHODS

Descriptive qualitative data, often seen in surveys, observational studies and case studies, is also known as categorical data, which is data that can be arranged categorically based on the qualities and characteristics of an event or a phenomenon being studied.[4] Categorical variables are defined as nominal, dichotomous or ordinal. Nominal variables describe categories that do not have a specific order to them such as ethnicity or gender. Dichotomous variables are categorical variables with two levels. These may include a yes/no or male/female response. Ordinal variables are generally subjective. They have two or more categories that can be ordered or ranked. For example, a response that ranges from strongly disagree to strongly agree would be considered ordinal. Similarly, researchers may sometimes consider ordinal variables as continuous if they have more than five categories.[4]

Qualitative data, on the other hand, used in qualitative methods such as ethnography, narrative, phenomenological, grounded theory and case study, are often similar in collection methods. Though similar, the use of textual or visual data is often differentiated by the aim of the study.[5] Qualitative data is typically ethnographic and interpretive; data is collected through direct or indirect participant observation or by asking open-ended questions. Popular qualitative collection methods include the following.

- *Participant observation:* The researcher is engaged in the group for some time. The behaviour of the group is explored by observing conversations and partaking in conversations with the group while taking field notes.

- *Interviews:* The researcher collects data directly from the interviewee on a one-to-one basis. The interview may be informal and unstructured or conversational. Mostly the open-ended questions are asked spontaneously. One-to-one interviews are particularly ideal when exploring sensitive topics. They provide rich and meaningful data while offering a safe environment that is sensitive to the participants' needs.

- *Focus groups:* A group discussion setting. The group is limited to 6 to 10 individuals who are purposely selected rather than from a statistically representative sample of a broader population. A moderator is assigned to moderate the ongoing discussion.
- *Document or artefact review:* This may be in the form of existing documents (government reports, documents, grey literature), field notes, photographs, videos or websites.

We have identified the different data types in qualitative research, we will now look at the specific qualitative methodologies and the data collected.

Ethnographic data collection is characterised by participant observation, where the researcher spends an extended period in a social group to collect data. It includes a collection of different ways of eliciting and collecting data, including the observation of individuals and groups of individuals, unstructured interviews, document analysis and the use of a researcher's field notes.[6] The researcher is the primary instrument for data collection and analysis. The researcher seeks to place specific events into a meaningful context, with a focus on the culture and social interaction of the participants or group.[6] Ethnography is specifically valuable in understanding the influence of social and cultural norms on the effectiveness of health interventions.[6,7]

Narrative approaches construct a sequence of events normally from one or two participants to form a cohesive story. In-depth interviews are conducted over time and presented as a story with themes. Intrinsic to narrative inquiry are the facets or faces of stories that give meaning to people's lives; these stories can be regarded as a data source. Narrative data is far more than the uncritical gathering of stories; using written, oral or visual narrative, it seeks to provide personal insight into the complexity of personal experiences.[8] Gare described storytelling as a primordial act of human existence and communication.[9] The stories we tell provide our identity, purpose and meaning; furthermore, stories convey our fears, hopes, cultural values and describe our 'lived time'.

Phenomenology seeks to study human experience and of the way things present themselves to us in and through our experience.[10] A combination of methods are used to collect data, such as conducting interviews, reading documents, watching videos or visiting places to form an understanding of the meaning participants place on the topic being researched. Similarly, grounded theory uses both extant and elicited data to build a theory based on the data. While interviews and document analysis are common, data sources often include focus groups, questionnaires, surveys, transcripts, letters, government reports, documents, grey literature, music, artefacts, videos, blogs and memos.[11]

Finally, a case study is described as a comprehensive systematic investigation of a single individual, group, community or some other unit in which the researcher studies in-depth data relating to several variables.[12] To begin, a single case or group of similar cases that can then be incorporated into a multiple-case study are specified, a review of what is known about the case(s) is conducted. This may include reviewing the literature, grey literature, media or reports. This data assists to establish a basic understanding of the cases and informs the research questions. Data in case studies are often, but not exclusively, qualitative.

CONCLUSION

This chapter identified types of qualitative data used in qualitative research methods. The non-numerical data is used to understand thoughts, concepts and experiences. Qualitative data enables the researcher to gain a deep insight into a research topic or phenomenon being studied. Qualitative data is important because it can examine the behaviour of people using a subjective method. Equally, it can also explore meaning and develop new theories that can be researched further.

REVIEW QUESTIONS

1. Describe sampling collection techniques included in qualitative research design.
2. Discuss the elements of structured and unstructured observational methods used in data collection.

SUGGESTED READING

Fry M, Curtis K, Considine J, Shaban RZ. Using observation to collect data in emergency research. Australasian Emergency Nursing Journal. 2017;20(1):25–30. Online. Available: http://doi.org/10.1016/j.aenj.2017.01.001.

Gibbs L, Kealy M, Willis K, Green J, Welch N, Daly J. What have sampling and data collection got to do with good qualitative research? Australian and New Zealand Journal of Public Health. 2007;31(6):540–544. Online. Available: http://doi.org/10.1111/j.1753–6405.2007.00140.x.

Palinkas LA, Horwitz SM, Green CA, Wisdom JP, Duan N, Hoagwood K. Purposeful sampling for qualitative data collection and analysis in mixed method implementation research. Administration and Policy in Mental Health and Mental Health Services Research. 2015;42(5):533–544. Online. Available: http://doi.org/10.1007/s10488-013-0528-y.

REFERENCES

1. Sandelowski M. Whatever happened to qualitative description? Research in Nursing & Health. Aug 2000;23(4):334–40.

Online. Available: http://doi.org/10.1002/1098-240x(200008)23:4<334::aid-nur9>3.0.co;2-g.

2. Nassaji H. Qualitative and descriptive research: data type versus data analysis. Language Teaching Research. 2015; 19(2):129–32. Online. Available: http://doi.org/10.1177/1362168815572747.

3. Hancock B, Ockleford E, Windridge K. An introduction to qualitative research. National Institute for Health Research, Yorkshire, UK; 2007.

4. Mackridge A, Rowe P. A practical approach to using statistics in health research: from planning to reporting. Newark, United States: John Wiley & Sons; 2018.

5. Creswell JW. Qualitative inquiry & research design: choosing among five approaches. Thousand Oaks, CA: Sage; 2007.

6. Morgan-Trimmer S, Wood F. Ethnographic methods for process evaluations of complex health behaviour interventions. Trials. 2016 2016/05/04;17(1):232. Online. Available: http://doi.org/10.1186/s13063-016-1340-2.

7. Curry LA, Nembhard IM, Bradley EH. Qualitative and mixed methods provide unique contributions to outcomes research.

2009;119(10):1442–52. Online. Available: http://doi.org/10.1161/CIRCULATIONAHA.107.742775.

8. Josselson R. The ethical attitude in narrative research: principles and practicalities. In: Clandinin DJ, editor. Handbook of narrative inquiry: mapping a methodology. London: SAGE Publications; 2007.

9. Gare A. The primordial role of stories in human self-creation. Cosmos and history. The Journal of Natural and Social Philosophy. 2007;3(1):93–114.

10. Gallagher S. What is phenomenology? In: Gallagher S, editor. Phenomenology. London: Palgrave Macmillan UK; 2012. pp. 7–18.

11. Chun Tie Y, Birks M, Francis K. Grounded theory research: a design framework for novice researchers. SAGE Open Med. 2019;7:2050312118822927. Online. Available: http://doi.org/10.1177/2050312118822927.

12. Heale R, Twycross A. What is a case study? Evidence-Based Nursing. 2018;21(1):7. Online. Available: http://doi.org/10.1136/eb-2017-102845.

43

Developing Themes

Belinda Flanagan

LEARNING OUTCOMES

1. Describe the meaning of thematic analysis
2. Recall the steps to conducting a thematic analysis, while differentiating codes and themes
3. Identify best practices in conducting a thematic analysis

INTRODUCTION

Methods for the analysis of qualitative data primarily involve formatting, condensing, arranging and constructing data codes, categories, themes and narratives.[1] To gain a comprehensive representation of the population or phenomenon being studied, the process of continuous sampling persists until saturation occurs, or no substantive new information is acquired.[2]

Thematic analysis as an independent qualitative descriptive approach is described as 'a method for identifying, analysing and reporting patterns (themes) within data'.[3] Braun and Clarke propose thematic analysis, which is a flexible and useful research tool that provides a rich and detailed, yet complex, account of the data.[3] Thematic analysis has also been described as a non-linear, iterative process, identifying common threads that extend across a dataset and providing a purely qualitative, detailed and nuanced account of the data.[3,4]

The current application of thematic analysis is associated with two modalities: inductive or deductive analysis. Inductive thematic analysis is used in cases where no previous studies researched the phenomenon, and therefore the coded categories are derived directly from the text data.[5] A deductive approach is useful if the general aim of thematic analysis is to test a previous theory in a different situation or to compare categories at different periods.[5] Regardless of the modality, the principles of thematic analysis—how to code data, refine themes and report findings—apply to several qualitative methods such as grounded theory, narrative or discourse analysis. Thematic analysis is a suitable

and robust method to use when seeking to understand a set of experiences, thoughts or behaviours across a dataset.[6]

STEPS TO THEMATIC ANALYSIS

Various methods can be used to form the categories with which thematic analysis can be conducted, ranging from creating the categories inductively using the data to creating the categories deductively based on an underlying theory from the field or the research question.[7] In most cases a multistage process of categorising and coding occurs, with the first phase identifying major themes and then a second phase detailing a more in depth approach where the categories are established and differentiated based on the data.[7] The significance of structuring data analysis in steps or phases is that it creates a transparent process for both the qualitative researcher and the reader of a thesis or publication. The following description of phases or steps to undertake a thematic analysis is based on Braun and Clarke's six steps of thematic analysis (see Fig 43.1).[3]

Step 1: Familiarising Yourself With the Data

This involves gathering all the audio or video interview files into one location, converting observational/field notes or memos to electronic format and scanning documents retrieved in paper form. Lester and colleagues recommend a structured naming protocol for each file, as well as the construction of a master data catalogue that lists each data source, its storage location, its creator and the date of its collection.[8] This step also includes careful and repeated active reading of the data text and highlighting important

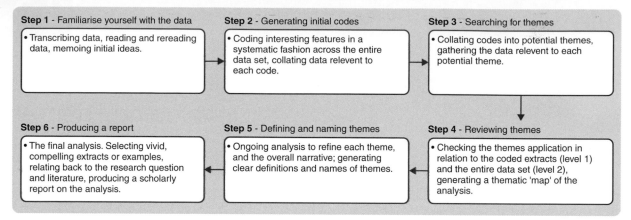

Figure 43.1 Braun and Clarke's six steps for thematic analysis. (Source: Braun V, Clarke V. Using thematic analysis in psychology. Qualitative Research in Psychology. 2006;3(2):77–101.)

passages or phrases. You may also add memos to the margins of the text of things that are relevant or interesting. Using voice recognition software or a transcription service is recommended. Familiarity with the data occurs as you check for accuracy.[6]

Step 2: Generating Initial Codes

This step includes the initial analysis of the data. From your notes or memos from step 1, start to make connections and form preliminary ideas and questions. This phase is purely about generating codes, not themes. A code is the most basic element of the raw data; it may be a word or short phrase that is symbolic for a portion of text or visual data.[9] A code sits within a larger coding framework. Deductive coding means you are starting with a predefined set of codes, then assigning them to the new data. These may come from previous research or literature. Inductive coding starts from the beginning and codes arise directly from the data.[6] Once the codes are created, the coding framework represents the organisation of the themes. There are normally two types: a flat coding frame or a hierarchical coding frame. A flat coding frame assigns the same level of importance to each code, whereas a hierarchical frame organises codes based on how they relate to each other.

Coding Methods

Coding can occur manually or with the assistance of computer software and should occur in at least two or more cycles. In inductive coding, the first coding cycle uses the participants' language, whereas the second coding cycle becomes more researcher-centric in the sense that concepts, themes and features from existing theories may be

presented.[9] In the first coding cycle, two types of codes are important: descriptive codes and attribute codes. Descriptive codes are assigned to sections of data based on what the section 'is about'. Sections of data are thus condensed using a label that specifies the meaning of the section of data concerning the overall research topic.[9]

Attribute codes are basic information assigned to large segments of data, typically to the units during which the data were originally collected like interviews, sites of observation or data sets.[9] Attribute codes assist to develop the coding framework and give structure to the dataset.[9] Codes develop from the first cycle of coding to the second cycle, and during the second cycle of coding the data requires 'classifying, prioritising, integrating, synthesising, abstracting and conceptualising, and theory building'.[10] The second phase of coding aims to connect statements, experiences and reflections offered by research participants.[8] As the research process develops, so does the type of coding, which also allows the researcher to move from basic descriptive codes towards answering the research question.[9]

Step 3: Searching for Themes

This step involves the examination of the codes to identify themes of significance.[3] According to Varpio and colleagues, themes do not emerge from the data; they are constructed by the researcher through analysing, comparing and graphically mapping how codes relate to each other.[11] Braun and Clarke described that in inductive analysis, the researcher derives themes from the coded data, so the themes identified will be more closely linked to the original data and reflective of the entire dataset.[3] Equally, in deductive analysis predefined theories and/or theoretical frameworks will advise theme development, so these themes focus on a particular aspect of the dataset or a specific question of interest.[3] When creating and organising themes, thematic maps are beneficial for visually demonstrating connections between concepts and among main themes and subthemes.[3]

Step 4: Reviewing Themes

Braun and Clarke described step 4 as a two-level analytical process.[3] In the first level of analysis, the researcher considers the coded data located within each theme to confirm they represent the theme accurately. Further sorting and adjustments can occur to better reflect the data. To validate rigour in the research process, detailed notes or memos should be kept demonstrating how themes were developed, removed and modified. Having an audit trail that describes the coding and analysis process will allow for transparency and reliability of the findings.[10] Level two similarly reviews the individual themes to ensure they fit within the dataset and that the thematic map accurately represents the entire body of data and illustrates the relationships between themes.[3]

Step 5: Defining and Naming Themes

Step 5 involves the researcher creating a definition and narrative description of each theme, including why it is significant to the broader research question.[3] This includes identifying important aspects of each theme and which aspects of the dataset it encompasses, creating a clear narrative of how and why the coded data within each theme contribute to the overall understanding of the research question.[3]

Step 6: Producing the Report/Manuscript

This final step involves writing up the ultimate analysis and outline of findings.[3] The final report should present a narrative that provides a clear and concise account of how the data was interpreted and why themes and interpretation of the data are important.[3] Narrative descriptions and representative data extracts (e.g. direct quotations from participants), should be used to describe the data as it offers notable answers to the research question.[3] Providing adequate context for data extracts is helpful to understand their importance.[3] The discussion section can broaden the analysis by relating themes to other literature, considering the implications of the findings and questioning the assumptions that gave rise to the themes.[3]

LIMITATIONS OF THEMATIC ANALYSIS

Braun and Clarke[3] discussed several limitations to avoid when conducting a thematic analysis. The first is a failure to adequately describe the assumptions that underlie the analysis. Whether the researcher used inductive or deductive analysis should be explicit and the analysis must align to those foundations.[3] The second is a lack of adequate analysis.[3] Interpretation of the data is important; merely providing data extracts does not constitute a thematic analysis. Braun and Clarke provided an example of how interview questions should not be used as themes as this shows a lack of analysis across the dataset.[3] The third is a weak analysis, where the claims or conclusions made in the report of findings are unsubstantiated.[3] Stating themes and extracts that are unsupported or contradicted by the data, this can be avoided by following the six-step method which contains built-in mechanisms for checking for internal consistency.[3]

CONCLUSION

Thematic analysis is the most common form of analysis in qualitative research. This type of analysis aptly identifies patterns within and across data sets that are important to describe a phenomenon and address a specific research question. Caution should be taken to ensure the coding that occurs identifies meaning-based patterns rather than a feature of the data. It is important to keep in mind when undertaking this type of analysis that themes **do not emerge**, they are conceptualised and represent the view of the participants.

REVIEW QUESTIONS

1. What types of results or findings are likely to be yielded from thematic analysis?
2. Which step of performing a thematic analysis concerns you the most as a researcher?
3. What steps are to be taken to add reliability and validity to a thematic analysis?

SUGGESTED READING

Bazeley P. Analysing qualitative data: more than 'identifying themes'. Malaysian Journal of Qualitative Research. 2009;2(2):6–22. Online. Available: http://www.researchsupport.com.au/Bazeley_MJQR_2009.pdf.

Hutchison AJ, Johnston LH, Breckon JD. Using QSR-NVivo to facilitate the development of a grounded theory project: an account of a worked example. International Journal of Social Research Methodology. 2010;13(4):283–302. Online. Available: http://doi.org/10.1080/13645570902996301.

Lacey A, Luff D. Qualitative research analysis. The NIHR RDS for the East Midlands/Yorkshire & the Humber; 2007, updated 2009. Online. Available: https://www.rds-yh.nihr.ac.uk/wp-content/uploads/2013/05/9_Qualitative_Data_Analysis_Revision_2009.pdf.

REFERENCES

1. Saldaña J. Introduction: Thinking about thinking. Thinking qualitatively; methods of mind. London: SAGE; 2015.
2. Palinkas LA, Horwitz SM, Green CA, Wisdom JP, Duan N, Hoagwood K. Purposeful sampling for qualitative data collection and analysis in mixed method implementation research. Administration and Policy in Mental Health. 2015;42(5):533–44.
3. Braun V, Clarke V. Using thematic analysis in psychology. Qualitative Research in Psychology. 2006;3(2):77–101.
4. DeSantis L, Ugarriza DN. The concept of theme as used in qualitative nursing research. Western Journal of Nursing Research. 2000;22(3):351–72.
5. Hsieh HF, Shannon SE. Three approaches to qualitative content analysis. Qualitative Health Research. 2005;15(9):1277–88.
6. Kiger ME, Varpio L. Thematic analysis of qualitative data: AMEE Guide No. 131. Medical Teacher. 2020;42(8):846–54.
7. Kuckartz U. Qualitative text analysis: a guide to methods, practice & using software. London: SAGE Publications Ltd; 2014. Available: https://methods.sagepub.com/book/qualitative-text-analysis.
8. Lester JN, Cho Y, Lochmiller CR. Learning to do qualitative data analysis: a starting point. Human Resource Development Review. 2020;19(1):94–106.
9. Skjott Linneberg M, Korsgaard S. Coding qualitative data: a synthesis guiding the novice. Qualitative Research Journal. 2019;19(3):259–70.
10. Saldana, J. Coding manual for qualitative researchers. 4th ed. Sage Publishing; 2021.
11. Varpio L, Ajjawi R, Monrouxe LV, O'Brien BC, Rees CE. Shedding the cobra effect: problematising thematic emergence, triangulation, saturation and member checking. Medical Education. 2017;51(1):40–50.

Other Ways to Answer the Question

Having explored what is available in the literature to date (Section 2, Part 3) and assessing the methodological considerations (Section 2, Part 4), given your specific study type you may find that neither a quantitative (Section 3) or qualitative (Section 4) approach is optimally suited for your research question or circumstances. Fortunately, there are other ways to answer the question.

Mixed methodology design (Chapter 44) integrates the best of quantitative and qualitative approaches into one research design and can help paint a more comprehensive picture. And although mixed methods research is relatively new and resource-intensive, the results obtained may provide meaningful contributions. While expert opinion ranks at the bottom of the evidence hierarchy, when the expertise and opinion of a group of experts are collected and analysed in a formal way—such as in a Delphi study (Chapter 45) or nominal group technique (Chapter 46)—they can be a cost-effective, rapid and suitable alterative for many research questions.

Lastly, because all resources are limited, the question of appropriate allocation emerges. Analysing how much return we get on any particular investment is therefore crucial and is the primary aim of cost–benefit and cost effectiveness research designs (Chapter 47).

44

Mixed Methods Design

Natalie Anderson

LEARNING OUTCOMES

1. Define mixed methods research design
2. Outline three major types of mixed methods designs
3. Identify the strengths and weaknesses of mixed methods designs
4. Describe how mixed methods are relevant and applicable to paramedicine research

DEFINITION

There is a lack of consensus on a single definition of mixed methods, but mixed methods research designs always involve the collection, analysis and integration of both qualitative and quantitative data.[1,2] The combination of research approaches can help to increase the breadth or depth of understandings.[3] For example, a research group in the United Kingdom used a mixed methods design to explore different measures of ambulance care.[4] Traditionally, ambulance services measure the speed of response and outcomes for select emergency conditions, but these may not be the only important performance indicators. The research project analysed a large case-matched dataset and sought perspectives from service leaders, paramedics and patients. Outcomes like survival and timely response are essential, but the study noted that other vital measures of quality—including the provision of effective pain management, reassurance for caregivers and patient education—were not routinely evaluated.

INTRODUCTION

When assessing patients, paramedics often collect, analyse and combine quantitative numerical data (e.g. blood pressure, heart rate, body temperature) and qualitative meaning-based data (e.g. patient symptoms, medical history, social support systems). Experienced paramedics know the value of integrating objective numerical recordings and more contextual and subjective qualitative findings when forming an overall clinical impression.

Just as paramedic work has moved from rigid algorithmic protocols to more discretionary and context-specific decision-making, paramedicine research designs are also evolving to explore complex clinical problems.[5] Although mixed methods studies make up only a small portion of currently published healthcare peer-reviewed research,[6] the use of mixed methods is increasingly popular in paramedicine research.[7] This fits well with a pragmatic researcher world view.[8] Biomedically focused clinical research provides valid, reliable evidence vital for clinical care. Well-designed quantitative studies can tell us which intervention works best overall, or which patient groups are most at risk of adverse health outcomes. Mixed methods designs can often provide a more in-depth, holistic view of patient or paramedic experiences or behaviour by including qualitative data. Sometimes this also explains *why* one intervention works better than another or identifies barriers and facilitators to quality healthcare provision.

MIXED METHODS DESIGN IN PARAMEDICINE RESEARCH

Mixed methods designs can take many forms. Qualitative and quantitative data can be collected concurrently (at the same time) or sequentially (in phases).[2] One methodology (qualitative or quantitative) may be prioritised, although paramedicine research often gives equal weighting to both data sources.[7] As described by Creswell and Clark,[2] the three core types of mixed methods research are presented in Figure 44.1 and outlined below with illustrative paramedic and prehospital research examples. These are simple key approaches, but large-scale mixed methods research can involve multiple phases, nested studies and other complex designs.

Convergent Design

Convergent designs can be the simplest and least resource-intensive mixed methods designs. Researchers merge findings from two complementary data sets that are collected at the same time. Quantitative and qualitative data are gathered and analysed concurrently, then combined and compared. It is important that the process of integrating data is clearly outlined and rationalised, to move beyond merely mixing data types, to quality mixed methods design. In many instances, the quantitative and qualitative data results complement each other and provide a richer picture of the topic being investigated.

A convergent mixed method design was used by Brett and colleagues to understand the psychological impact of COVID-19 on paramedic students.[9] Quantitative data arising from a self-report measure provided insights into student anxiety levels. Qualitative semi-structured interviews identified students' key stressors and coping strategies.

Explanatory Sequential Design

An explanatory sequential design helps researchers to explain a phenomenon and answer questions about why or how that phenomenon presents. This approach usually consists of an initial, major quantitative data collection phase, such as a large survey of patient perceptions of paramedic practitioner care. This would then be followed by a smaller qualitative study; for example, patient focus groups discussing experiences of paramedic practitioner care. Curtis and colleagues used an explanatory sequential study design to understand the impact of a trial of prehospital blood collection.[10] During the trial, paramedics were supported to take blood samples when canulating patients. Researchers used a retrospective controlled cohort study to determine how this impacted the time taken for available results, labelling errors and haemolysis rates. They then surveyed local paramedics, using open-ended questions to assess their perceptions of prehospital blood collection and identify any barriers and facilitators.

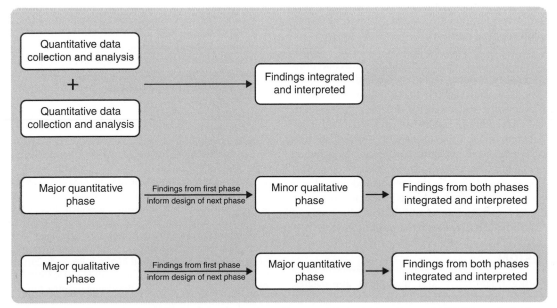

Figure 44.1 Core mixed methods research designs. (Source: Adapted from Creswell JW, Plano Clark VL. Designing and conducting mixed methods research. 3rd ed. Sage Publications; 2017.)

Exploratory Sequential Design

Exploratory sequential designs are often used when little is known about a new or complex phenomenon. For example: Why do older adults sometimes delay calling an ambulance? How do patients who have self-harmed experience emergency ambulance care? How do paramedics make sense of ethically challenging situations?

Exploratory sequential designs begin with the collection and analysis of qualitative data. The qualitative phase helps explore the area and may identify key factors, a model or theory that can then be tested in a quantitative phase. Anderson and colleagues used an exploratory sequential research design to explore paramedic decisions to start, continue or stop resuscitation.[11] Their research began with qualitative in-depth interviews, followed by focus groups and finally a quantitative survey of paramedic students. Findings were integrated to develop a model of prehospital resuscitation decision-making which incorporated paramedic experiences, preparation and support.

STRENGTHS AND WEAKNESSES

Because mixed methods designs are relatively new to the paramedic discipline, proving the reliability, trustworthiness, quality and rigour of studies can be more challenging. High-quality mixed methods research designs provide a clear rationale for gathering both qualitative and quantitative data. The types of data collected, methods of collection and sequencing of when data is collected must be clearly outlined. Integration of the qualitative and quantitative data should be underpinned by a clear theoretical framework or philosophical position.

Mixed methods research designs have several inherent strengths and weaknesses. By using multiple data collections and combining approaches (quantitative and qualitative), mixed methods research can help to offset the weaknesses of each. However, some argue that the different philosophical worldviews underpinning qualitative and quantitative research are incompatible. Other challenges in mixed methods designs include the need for significant resources, including time for sequential research designs. Members of the research team also need to have diverse methodological and data analysis skillsets. Mixed methods research can also be challenging to report succinctly, and difficulties can arise if quantitative and qualitative findings are contradictory.

CONCLUSION

By integrating quantitative and qualitative approaches, mixed methods research designs can help to comprehensively examine complex problems in paramedicine practice and education. Although combining both approaches can offer 'the best of both worlds', mixed methods research designs can be resource-intensive and present some methodological challenges. However, the results obtained by using both research design approaches are often richer, are more relevant to patient care and make a meaningful contribution to the body of paramedicine empirical knowledge and evidence.

REVIEW QUESTIONS

1. What is mixed methods research design?
2. What research questions in paramedicine could be addressed by mixed methods research designs?
3. What challenges might paramedicine researchers face if they choose to undertake a mixed methods research design?

REFERENCES

1. Curry LA, Nunez-Smith M. Mixed methods in health sciences research: a practical primer. SAGE Publications; 2015. Online. Available: https://doi.org/10.4135/9781483390659.
2. Creswell JW, Plano Clark VL. Designing and conducting mixed methods research. 3rd ed. Sage Publications; 2017.
3. Johnson RB, Onwuegbuzie AJ, Turner LA. Toward a definition of mixed methods research. Journal of Mixed Methods Research. 2007;1(2):112–33. Online. Available: https://doi.org/10.1177/1558689806298224.
4. Turner J, Siriwardena AN, Coster J, Jacques R, Irving AS, Crum A, et al. Developing new ways of measuring the quality and impact of ambulance service care: the PhOEBE mixed-methods research programme. Programme Grants for Applied Research. 2019;7(3). Online. Available: https://doi.org/10.3310/pgfar07030.
5. Whitley GA, Munro S, Hemingway P, Law GR, Siriwardena AN, Cooke D, et al. Mixed methods in pre-hospital research: Understanding complex clinical problems. British Paramedic Journal. 2020;5(3):44–51. Online. Available: https://doi.org/10.29045/14784726.2020.12.5.3.44.
6. Wisdom JP, Cavaleri MA, Onwuegbuzie AJ, Green CA. Methodological reporting in qualitative, quantitative and mixed methods health services research articles. Health Services Research, 2012;47(2):721–45. Online. Available: https://doi.org/10.1111/j.1475–6773.2011.01344.x.
7. McManamny T, Sheen J, Boyd L, Jennings PA. Mixed methods and its application in prehospital research: A systematic review. Journal of Mixed Methods Research. 2015;9(3):214–31. Online. Available: https://doi.org/10.1177/1558689813520408.
8. Feilzer MY. Doing mixed methods research pragmatically: implications for the rediscovery of pragmatism as a research paradigm. Journal of Mixed Methods Research. 2010;4(1):6–16. Online. Available: https://doi.org/10.1177/1558689809349691.
9. Brett W, King C, Shannon B, Gosling C. Impact of COVID-19 on paramedicine students: A mixed methods study. International Emergency Nursing. 2021;56:100996. Online. Available: https://doi.org/10.1016/j.ienj.2021.100996.

10. Curtis K, Ellwood J, Walker A, Qian S, Delamont P, Yu P, et al. Implementation evaluation of pre-hospital blood collection in regional Australia: a mixed methods study. Australasian Emergency Care. 2021:24(4):255–63. Online. Available: https://doi.org/10.1016/j.auec.2020.08.007.

11. Anderson NE, Slark J, Gott M. Prehospital resuscitation decision-making: a model of ambulance personnel experiences, preparation and support. Emergency Medicine Australasia. 2021;33:697–702. Online. Available: https://doi.org/10.1111/1742-6723.13715.

45

Consensus Group Methods— The Delphi Technique

Liam Langford

LEARNING OUTCOMES

1. Recognise the purpose of using consensus methods in research
2. Identify the strengths and weaknesses of Delphi Technique
3. Describe the process of the of the Delphi Technique

DEFINITION

The Delphi technique is a coordinated process for collating and synthesising knowledge from expert panellists through rounds of anonymised opinions and questionnaires.[1]

INTRODUCTION

As the name alludes to, consensus group methods are as a systematic means for measuring and developing consensus. They are mostly used in conditions where there is uncertainty, conflict or incomplete evidence. Usually, groups comprise of experts relevant to the study aim. Of the consensus group methods, the Delphi technique is most widely used.[2]

Originally developed in the 1950s by the RAND Corporation to predict the impact of technology on warfare, the Delphi technique has been extensively used across disciplines to assist with creating consensus, group judgments and informing decisions.[3] Rounds, consisting of a qualitative, quantitative or combination of questionnaires, are conducted until a consensus is achieved among the expert panellists. During the process panellists are unaware of one another and never interact. At this stage, there is no exact gold standard reporting guideline for Delphi studies and, over time, variations to the process have evolved to meet research needs.

STRENGTHS OF THE DELPHI TECHNIQUE

The Delphi technique has a number of strengths that can assist researchers in designing, collaborating and implementing the method relevant to their research question.[4,5] The Delphi technique's design can be simple and flexible. Depending on the question and purpose it can be qualitative, quantitative or mixed methods. Additionally, the Delphi technique enables access to experts and their insights, while potentially causing them to evaluate their opinions and learn/develop new knowledge. Given their involvement, experts are more likely to accept results and aid in dissemination. When conducting a Delphi technique, the response rates are generally high, with the anonymity and democratic aspects mitigating individuals influencing group dynamics and biasing outcomes. Furthermore, the Delphi technique is a relatively cost-effective method, especially when conducted electronically.

WEAKNESSES OF THE DELPHI TECHNIQUE

There are, however, some drawbacks and critiques of the Delphi Technique.[4,5] For a consensus method, there appears to be little consensus on terminology, design and parameters. Often researchers will conduct a 'modified' Delphi technique, despite high ambiguity of its nature and term. Furthermore, there is significant variation and debate in prescribed panel size, consensus levels, rounds and overall approach. Therefore, researchers must be robust in their justification for decisions and variations. From some scholars' aspects, the Delphi technique is not considered a valid scientific method nor is its theoretical basis well established. It is also asserted that the approach to communication is restrictive and does not facilitate debate and problem identification. Outcomes may also be a result of collective ignorance as opposed to collective wisdom.

When conducting the method, it has been noted that inappropriate expert selection can occur, leading to muddled results. Furthermore, timelines can become protracted if multiple rounds are required due to disagreements. This protraction also increases the risk of participant attrition.

THE DELPHI TECHNIQUE PROCESS

Justification

It is imperative that the aim of the research aligns with the Delphi techniques strengths (refer to above). Additionally, the Delphi technique method can be used when there is limited or conflicting information or for developing new concepts, decision-making and/or agenda setting.[6]

Establish Expert Panellists Criteria and Sampling

The Delphi technique is not concerned with a generalised sample population, but a purposive sample of individuals with expertise on a given topic.[7] However, there is no consensus on what constitutes an expert.[5] The inclusion criteria of what defines an expert for the study is usually decided by the steering research group.[8] Once established, sampling can occur via direct communication or a snowball technique. To ensure rigor and trustworthiness, the criteria and sampling strategy have to be reported.

Determine Size of Panel

There is no set size required for a panel; however, six experts have been considered the minimum requirement. It is common to have between 10 and 20 panellists. While there may be a sense that increasing the size of the panel thereby increases the validity, it can make the process unstable and time consuming. Consideration and justification of panel size needs to support the aim of the research and be appropriately reported.[6]

Confirm Consensus

There is no set definition or criteria for consensus in the Delphi technique.[9] This is determined by the authors or the steering research group before the study begins. Most studies have used a percentage of agreement (mainly 75% or 80%), median score or a combination of both.[6] Consensus, however defined by researchers, should be justified and reported.

Questionnaire Design

Questionnaire design depends on the aim of the research and preexisting information. It can use both quantitative and qualitative methods. As an example, researchers may develop a Likert-scale questionnaire informed by systematic or literature reviews, a synthesis of already existing guidelines or from a conceptual framework.[6] Seven-point Likert scales are considered accurate in measuring a participant's true evaluation.[10]

The first round can be unstructured or semi-structured with open questions. This promotes participants' relative freedom and scope to elaborate on the subject being investigated. Alternatively, a quantitative questionnaire can be derived from a literature review.[1]

Analysis

A qualitative analysis (e.g. thematic analysis) of the results is then undertaken. This creates a foundation to construct the second and subsequent questionnaires.[1] Any qualitative analysis method should aim to limit bias and should be included in the final report. If questionnaires are designed with the Likert scale or other quantitative methods, appropriate analysis must be used.

Number of Rounds

As with other aspects of the Delphi technique, there are no hard guidelines for the number of rounds.[8] It depends on when consensus is met. Most studies have two to three rounds until consensus is achieved; however, others have been known to achieve consensus with five or more rounds. Increasing the number of rounds can have consequences. Consensus may have been as a result of survey fatigue. That is, participants may not hold a consensus view, but to finish lengthy and numerous rounds participants may concede. Other issues arising from numerous rounds can include higher attrition rates and an increase in the length of the study period.[2]

Given these issues, some scholars state that the Delphi technique should be limited to no more than three rounds, and with the areas where no consensus was apparent, should also be reported. Either approach (continuous round until consensus or predetermined number) should be justified and reported.

Length of Rounds

The duration of a round once again depends on the context of the study. Usually, a round lasts 1 to 4 weeks, although there is a version of the Delphi technique that conducts a round in real-time.

Delphi Technique Process Flowchart

An overview of the Delphi technique's process is outlined below in Figure 45.1.

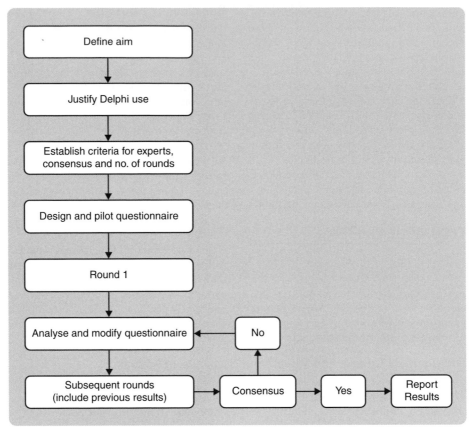

Figure 45.1 Delphi technique process flowchart

EXAMPLE

Jamie is a paramedic who has been tasked with developing a new paramedic educator role for their organisation. As this is a new role, there are no established capability frameworks that outline the skills, knowledge and attributes that the educators require. To guide the selection process of applicants, budget for their training needs and performance management system, Jamie will need to create a Paramedic Educator Capability Framework. Jamie can use the Delphi technique to facilitate structured dialogue, reduce bias and establish a consensus on the required capabilities for the paramedic educator role.

Jamie begins by establishing the research question and *aim*: 'What are the capabilities required for the role of a paramedic educator within the context of the organisation?'

As there are differing opinions and sporadic literature about what capabilities are required for the role and noting that accommodating travel and schedules of experts for face-to-face dialogue and meetings is unfeasible, Jamie can *justify* using the Delphi technique.

Jamie *establishes the criteria to be an expert panellist* to be paramedic manager or senior academic with more than 5 years' experience in health professional education. The *panel size* they are aiming for is a minimum six members and no more than 12. *Sampling* of panellists occurs from different networks and by reviewing authors from relevant research articles. A mix of internal, national and international experts are identified.

Based on other studies' *consensus* definition and criteria, Jamie decided that 80% of panellists will need to agree on each capability for it to be considered consensus.

As there is no previous research on the given area, Jamie will use an open-ended *questionnaire design* in the first round to elicit qualitative feedback. After analysis of the qualitative responses, they will design a Likert scale questionnaire with some limited free-text questions for subsequent rounds. Before dissemination, the questionnaires were tested with non-panellist colleagues. Table 45.1 outlines the how Jamie conducted their Delphi technique based on the established parameters and subsequent participants' input.

TABLE 45.1	**Jamie's Delphi Technique Process and Outcomes**
Round 1	In total, 11 invitations, details, deadlines and questionnaires have been sent to the identified experts. They are given 1 week to respond. Ten panellists complete and return the questionnaire.
Analysis	Jamie uses thematic analysis to identify possible capabilities and create the questionnaire for round 2 from the themes.
Round 2	The new questionnaire was distributed to the panellists and they were all completed and within 1 week.
Analysis	All capabilities except for one reached 80% agreement. This was sufficient for consensus and completion of the Delphi technique process. During reporting, Jamie will report on the capabilities that did not reach consensus.

CONCLUSION

Consensus methods such as the Delphi technique are useful research tools in paramedicine. They are flexible and require little resources. Additionally, they can help identify problems, prioritise actions, build a shared understanding and establish agreements. However, they do have their limitations. Thus their use must be justified appropriately and meet the aim of the study. Furthermore, modifications must be reported on.

REVIEW QUESTIONS

1. What is the purpose of using consensus methods in research?
2. Identify four strengths and four weaknesses of the Delphi technique.
3. Fill in the boxes of the flowchart to help describe the Delphi technique process.

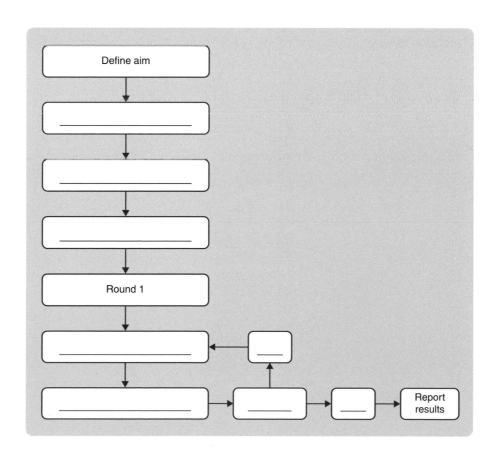

SUGGESTED FURTHER READING

Jünger S, Payne SA, Brine J, Radbruch L, Brearley SG. Guidance on Conducting and REporting DElphi Studies (CREDES) in palliative care: recommendations based on a methodological systematic review. Palliative Medicine. 2017;31(8):684–706.

Waggoner J, Carline JD, Durning SJ. Is there a consensus on consensus methodology? Descriptions and recommendations for future consensus research. Academic Medicine. 2016;91(5).

REFERENCES

1. Powell C. The Delphi technique: myths and realities. Journal of Advanced Nursing. 2003;41(4):376–82.

2. Humphrey-Murto S, Varpio L, Gonsalves, C, Wood TJ. Using consensus group methods such as Delphi and Nominal Group in medical education research. Medical Teacher. 2017;39(1):14–19. Online. Available: https://doi.org/10.1080/0142159X.2017.1245856.

3. The RAND Corporation. Delphi Method. RAND; 2016. Online. Available: https://www.rand.org/topics/delphi-method.html.

4. Hasson F, Keeney S. Enhancing rigour in the Delphi technique research. Technological Forecasting and Social Change. 2011;78(9):1695–704. Online. Available: https://doi.org/10.1016/j.techfore.2011.04.005.

5. Vernon W. The Delphi technique: a review. International Journal of Therapy and Rehabilitation. 2009;16(2):69–76.

6. Jünger S, Payne SA, Brine J, Radbruch L, Brearley SG. Guidance on Conducting and REporting DElphi Studies (CREDES) in palliative care: recommendations based on a methodological systematic review. Palliative Medicine. 2017;31(8):684–706. Online. Available: https://doi.org/10.1177/0269216317690685.

7. Keeney S, Hasson F, McKenna HP. A critical review of the Delphi technique as a research methodology for nursing. International Journal of Nursing Studies. 2001;38(2):195–200. Online. Available: https://doi.org/https://doi.org/10.1016/S0020-7489(00)00044-4

8. Foth T, Efstathiou N, Vanderspank-Wright B, Ufholz LA, Dütthorn N, Zimansky M, Humphrey-Murto S. The use of Delphi and Nominal Group Technique in nursing education: A review. International Journal of Nursing Studies. 2016;60:112–20. Online. Available: https://doi.org/10.1016/j.ijnurstu.2016.04.015.

9. Waggoner J, Carline JD, Durning SJ. Is there a consensus on consensus methodology? Descriptions and recommendations for future consensus research. Academic Medicine. 2016;91(5). Online. Available: https://journals.lww.com/academicmedicine/Fulltext/2016/05000/Is_There_a_Consensus_on_Consensus_Methodology_.22.aspx.

10. Finstad K. Response interpolation and scale sensitivity: Evidence against 5-point scales. Journal of Usability Studies. 2010;5(3):104–10.

46

Consensus Group Methods— The Nominal Group Technique

Liam Langford

LEARNING OUTCOMES

1. Recall why a researcher might use a nominal group technique
2. Identify the strengths and weaknesses of the nominal group technique
3. Describe the process of the nominal group technique

DEFINITION

The nominal group technique (NGT) is a 'structured, well-established, multistep, facilitated, group meeting technique used to generate and prioritise responses to a specific question by a group of people who have expert insight into a particular area of interest'.[1]

INTRODUCTION

Originally developed in the field of social psychology, the NGT has been used extensively in education and health. As an example, it has been useful in problem identification, solution development, action prioritisation, strategic direction creation, curriculum and clinical guideline design.[2] In paramedicine, the NGT has assisted to develop consensus education and clinical governance.[3,4] The traditional NGT consists of five phases: 1. introduction and explanation; 2. silent generation; 3. round robin; 4. discussion/clarification; and 5. ranking. (See Figure 46.1.)

STRENGTHS OF THE NOMINAL GROUP TECHNIQUE

There are several strengths of NGTs in research, depending on the research's purpose.[5,6] Rich data can emerge from lively discussion. These discussions can also develop collaborative relationships and shared mental models among participants. The participants can receive instantaneous feedback and results, which aids in creating a sense of reward and closure. From a resource perspective, NGTs are time efficient and require few outlays or upfront costs.

WEAKNESSES OF THE NOMINAL GROUP TECHNIQUE

Foth and colleagues and Humphrey-murto and colleagues highlight varying weakness of NGTs.[5,6] These include: critiques and apprehensions about its methodological rigor and trustworthiness; its ambiguous definitions of consensus and expert; its small sample size; and the influence of dominating participants on the group and bias outcomes.

NOMINAL GROUP TECHNIQUE PROCESS

The traditional NGT is comprised of five phases. However, some preparations are required before beginning the process.

- *Question development:* In the NGT, only one or two questions that are underpinned by the study aim are posed to the group. Any more questions and the process risks losing focus or becoming complex/confusing.
- *Group size and composition:* For the NGT, sizes have ranged from 2 to 14 people, but a maximum of seven is recommended.[7] Because NGT is face to face, composition is limited to the expert's availability. Selection of an expert is based on their expertise and their relevance to the study aim/questions. Non-experts can also be used, depending on their relevance to the aim.

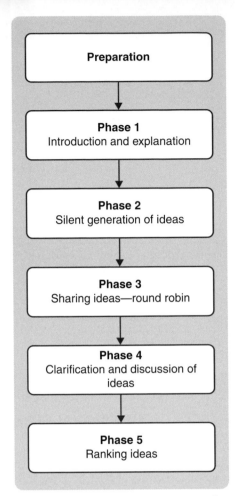

Figure 46.1 Nominal group technique process flowchart

Phase 2: Silent Generation of Ideas

In the silent generation phase, participants spend approximately 20 minutes pondering and/or recording their ideas and answers to the question(s). As per the name, there is no discussion or talking within this phase.

Phase 3: Sharing Ideas—Round Robin

For the 'round robin' phase, the facilitator asks participants one at a time to state their ideas and answers to the question(s). Observing participants can continue to generate ideas. The length of the phase depends on how long it takes for all ideas to be exhausted. No discussion or qualifiers to answers usually occur in the round robin. All ideas are recorded verbatim on a whiteboard or shared electronic document.

Phase 4: Discussion/Clarification of Ideas

The discussion and clarification phase ensures participants understand the meaning of individual ideas. Guided by the facilitator, participants could either take responses at face value or articulate the nuances of their responses. This would be done simultaneously when either condensing ideas into groups/themes and/or removing duplicates. This is usually the longest phase in the NGT, with the facilitator playing an important role in setting the pace and ensuring some participants do not dominate the group dynamics.

Phase 5: Ranking Ideas

After discussions, participants would then rank the ideas or issues. Depending on the group dynamics and aim of the study, this can be done anonymously or as a group. Methods for ranking could include from highest to lowest, top four or Likert scale. Re-ranking, after participants have viewed the first-round results, is also an option.[7]

EXAMPLE

Lindsey is a paramedic working in health policy. They have been tasked with investigating the incorporation of paramedics into palliative healthcare services. To identify the barriers and enablers to paramedics being incorporated into palliative healthcare services, Lindsey will use an NGT.

Preparing for the NGT, Lindsey does the following:
- clarifies the question they want to ask
- identifies and invites 8 to 12 relevant experts (clinicians, academics, managers and policy developers)
- enlists two facilitators
- chooses an appropriate venue and time for face-to-face interaction.

- *NGT facilitators:* NGT requires facilitators to coordinate and enact the phases. Usually, this is two to three facilitators per NGT, one to coordinate and the others to collect responses and transcribe them to a whiteboard or virtual shared document.[8] Ideally, facilitators have been trained or had previous experience with NGT.

Nominal Group Technique Phases
Phase 1: Introduction and Explanation

During phase 1, facilitators introduce themselves and the participants. They explain the purpose and process of the NGT to the group members/participants. Consent, in line with your ethics, may be gained prior to or during phase 1. Finally, the study's question(s) are posed to the group.

The NGT starts with Lindsey welcoming the expert participants, introducing them to each other, **explaining** the purpose and process of the NGT and providing them with the questions. The participants sit **silently generating** ideas to the questions. Some write them down. After 20 minutes, Lindsey begins the next phase.

In a **round-robin** fashion, they ask the participants to share one idea at a time. A facilitator records their ideas on sticky notes and adds them to the whiteboard. This continues until the participants do not generate any new ideas.

Lindsey now asks the panellists if they would like any ideas **clarified**, while grouping the ideas into similar themes. During this phase, one participant appears to be dominating the discussion. Lindsey recognises this, moderates the discussion and ensures other participants are included. After an hour or so, participants have now clarified points of terminology, organised ideas into themes and discarded any duplicates.

Participants are now asked to **rank** the top four barriers and enablers to paramedics being incorporated into palliative healthcare services. They do this anonymously on a ranking template. Lindsey checks the results and confirms there is consensus among the group. The results are shared with the group immediately.

For Lindsey, the barriers and enablers of incorporating paramedics into palliative healthcare services have now been identified. From here, Lindsey develops action items and works with stakeholders to overcome the barriers and enhance the enablers.

For the participants, they now have developed new networks with a shared understanding of the topic. The collegiality among the group assists Lindsey with policy implementation.

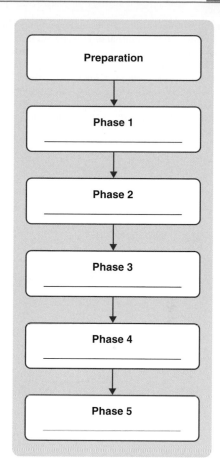

CONCLUSION

Consensus methods, such as the nominal group technique, are useful research tools in paramedicine. They are flexible and require little resources. Additionally, they can help identify problems, prioritise actions, build a shared understanding and establish agreements. However, consensus methods do have their limitations, so their use must be justified appropriately and meet the aim of the study. Furthermore, modifications must be reported.

REVIEW QUESTIONS

1. What uses does the NGT have in research?
2. Identify four strengths and four weaknesses of the NGT.
3. Fill in the boxes of the flowchart to help describe the NGT process.

REFERENCES

1. Søndergaard E, Ertmann RK, Reventlow S, Lykke K. Using a modified nominal group technique to develop general practice. BMC Family Practice. 2018;19(1):1–9. Online. Available: https://doi.org/10.1186/s12875-018-0811-9.
2. Harvey N, Holmes CA. Nominal group technique: an effective method for obtaining group consensus. International Journal of Nursing Practice. 2012;18(2):188–194. Online. Available: https://doi.org/https://doi.org/10.1111/j.1440-172X.2012.02017.x.
3. Barr N, Lane M, Lord B. Use of a nominal group technique to evaluate a remote area simulation event for paramedicine students. International Paramedic Practice. 2016;6(1):13–18.
4. Sunde GA, Kottmann A, Heltne J-K, Sandberg M, Gellerfors M, Krüger A, et al. Standardised data reporting from prehospital advanced airway management—a nominal group technique update of the Utstein-style airway template. Scandinavian Journal of Trauma, Resuscitation and Emergency Medicine. 2018;26(1):1–16.
5. Foth T, Efstathiou N, Vanderspank-Wright B, Ufholz LA, Dütthorn N, Zimansky M, Humphrey-Murto S. The use of

Delphi and Nominal Group Technique in nursing education: A review. International Journal of Nursing Studies. 2016; 60:112–20. Online. Available: https://doi.org/10.1016/j.ijnurstu.2016.04.015.

6. Humphrey-murto S, Varpio L, Gonsalves C, Wood TJ, Varpio L, Gonsalves C, Wood TJ. Using consensus group methods such as Delphi and Nominal Group in medical education research. Medical Teacher. 2017;39(1):14–19. Online. Available: https://doi.org/10.1080/0142159X.2017.1245856.

7. McMillan SS, Kelly F, Sav A, Kendall E, King MA, Whitty JA, Wheeler AJ. Using the Nominal Group Technique: how to analyse across multiple groups. Health Services and Outcomes Research Methodology. 2014;14(3):92–108. Online. Available: https://doi.org/10.1007/s10742-014-0121-1.

8. Carney O, McIntosh J, Worth A. The use of the Nominal Group Technique in research with community nurses. Journal of Advanced Nursing. 1996;23(5):1024–9. Online. Available: https://doi.org/10.1046/j.1365-2648.1996.09623.x.

47

Cost-Effectiveness Research

Jonathan Foo, You You, Kieran Walsh and Stephen Maloney

LEARNING OUTCOMES

1. Explain the benefit of economic evidence to paramedic practice
2. Describe the steps taken to conduct a cost-effectiveness analysis
3. Describe the strengths and weaknesses of cost-effectiveness analyses

INTRODUCTION

Healthcare resources—people, equipment and facilities—are limited. As a result, individuals, organisations and governments must make choices to adopt certain options while foregoing other alternatives.[1] Economics is the study of the optimal allocation of limited resources for the production of benefit to society and is therefore relevant to any healthcare decision.[2]

The purpose of this chapter is to provide a primer on key economic concepts and methods within the context of paramedicine research. This should enable readers to consider whether an economic element would enhance their research, conduct basic economic research, hold informed discussions with economic specialists and undertake further learning on more advanced economic topics.

Cost-effectiveness analyses (CEAs) are one of the most common types of economic evaluations. They combine outcomes data from traditional effectiveness research with cost, providing useful evidence on which to base resource allocation decisions. The next sections will first introduce the concept of cost then subsequently describe the steps taken in conducting a CEA. A running case study has been included to demonstrate the application of key concepts (Box 47.1).

STEPS REQUIRED TO CONDUCT YOUR OWN STUDY OF THIS DESIGN

Economic cost (also known as opportunity cost) is the value you give up when you choose one intervention over the next best alternative. It includes not only direct monetary transactions (e.g. payment of wages) and physical transfer of resources (e.g. application of first-aid products), but also the foregone opportunity to use a resource for other purposes (e.g. volunteer time).[3]

Costing involves the steps of identifying, measuring and valuing all resources consumed and involves the following steps.[4]

1. *Identifying*: The major resource items that will influence the decision-making process should be identified and included in the costing. This will be guided by the perspective of the analysis; that is, from whose point of view should costs be considered (e.g. health service, patient). Resources may be identified through document review (e.g. financial statements, process flowcharts), through surveys or interviews or by direct observation. Common types of resources include personnel (e.g. emergency department staffing), equipment and materials (e.g. ambulance), consumables (e.g. medicines), facilities and maintenance (e.g. community health site) and patient or community inputs (e.g. patient time).
2. *Measuring*: For each identified resource, the quantity of use should be measured in natural units. Measurement is a balance between accuracy and effort to measure, and should be influenced by the intended use of the results.[5] Measurement may involve primary sources (e.g. interviews, surveys) or secondary sources (e.g. electronic medical records, administrative billing systems).[3]

Government X has committed to reducing deaths from cardiac arrest in community sport. They are considering two interventions:
- AED group—automated external defibrillator (AED) installment and maintenance at match grounds
- CPR group—cardiopulmonary resuscitation (CPR) training for coaches and match officials.

A pilot study is conducted in 40 community sport clubs. Clubs are randomly allocated to an intervention after controlling for club characteristics. Survival rates from cardiac arrest are monitored over 5 years. You conduct a CEA from the perspective of Government X over a 5-year period.

3. *Valuing*: Each resource must be assigned a monetary value. Monetisation can be done using a market price, the price at which an item is bought or sold, if available (e.g. medicine valued at the retail price). Values for health conditions or procedures may also exist in certain health systems; for example, based on diagnostic-related groups or the International Classification of Disease (ICD).[5] For resources that are not commonly bought or sold (e.g. patient time), non-market valuation approaches such as willingness to pay may be used. Refer to Baker and Ruting for a primer on non-market valuation approaches.[6]

Finally, the cost of a resource is calculated by multiplying the quantity of consumption by the per unit value. This can be further transformed and expressed in various ways, such as cost per episode, cost per patient or total program cost. Refer to Table 47.1 for an example of the costing process based on the running case study.

COST-EFFECTIVENESS ANALYSES

CEAs measure costs and effects of a program compared to at least one alternative. Effects can be measured through normal quantitative designs (e.g. randomised controlled trials) and may include patient-reported experience and outcome measures, intermediate outcomes (e.g. ambulance response times) or health outcomes (e.g. mortality rate). Costs and effects are considered for each alternative relative to a baseline. This is calculated and reported as a fraction, with the difference in costs as the numerator and the difference in effects as the denominator: the incremental cost-effectiveness ratio (ICER).[7] Box 47.2 demonstrates the ICER calculation applied to the case study.

STRENGTHS AND WEAKNESSES OF THIS DESIGN

CEAs are most useful when decision-makers have a defined budget and want to select between alternatives. However, CEAs are not useful when there is no reasonable comparator, or when there is no single measure of effect that can be used to compare across interventions.[1] Cost–benefit analyses (CBAs) are an extension of the CEA, where effects are converted to monetary units. This allows an individual intervention to be evaluated without a comparator, aggregation of multiple outcomes and comparison across different sectors (e.g. health and education).[1]

CONCLUSION

CEAs are useful tools for supporting efficient use of available resources. Given the variety of methods, assumptions and value judgments inherent in healthcare research, researchers should aim to conduct and report their methodological choices in an explicit and transparent manner.[8] Ultimately, decisions should not be made on an economic basis alone. Decision-makers should also be mindful of a range of influences, including local contexts, organisational values and political factors.

TABLE 47.1   Case Study—Identifying, Measuring and Valuing Costs

Resource item	Quantity (*Q*)	Value (*V*)	Cost (*Q* × *V*)
AED devices	20 units *Source: Program documents*	$2,000 per unit; includes purchase and maintenance *Source: Advertised retail price*	$40,000
CPR instructor time	200 hours; includes initial training and refresher training *Source: Training schedule documents*	$70 per hour *Source: Paramedic collective workplace agreement*	$14,000
CPR manikins	10 units *Source: Program documents*	$700 per unit *Source: Advertised retail price*	$7,000

BOX 47.2 Case Study—Incremental Cost-Effectiveness Ratio

Without intervention (i.e. the baseline), there is a 10% survival rate at a cost of $0. For the AED intervention, there is a 35% survival rate at a cost of $40,000. For the CPR intervention there is a 15% survival rate at a cost of $21,000.

AED Compared to Baseline

$$\frac{\text{AED cost} - \text{baseline cost}}{\text{AED survival} - \text{baseline survival}} = \frac{40,000 - 0}{35\% - 10\%} = 1600$$

Interpretation: In the AED group, it costs $1600 to gain 1% in survival rate.

CPR Compared to Baseline

$$\frac{\text{CPR cost} - \text{baseline cost}}{\text{CPR survival} - \text{baseline survival}} = \frac{21,000 - 0}{15\% - 10\%} = 4200$$

Interpretation: In the CPR group, it costs $4200 to gain 1% in survival rate.

These results can be represented graphically on the cost-effectiveness plane (Figure 47.1). Relative to the origin, the quadrants represent options that are more effective and more costly (upper right), more effective and less costly (lower right), less effective and less costly (lower left) and less effective and more costly (upper left).

Case Study Conclusion

Both interventions were more effective and more costly than the baseline, illustrated by their position in the upper-right quadrant of the cost-effectiveness plane. The AED intervention is more cost-effective than CPR, illustrated by the smaller gradient of the line from the origin, costing $1600 per 1% gain in survival rate compared to $4200. If costs were also considered from the perspective of society as a whole, the time taken to train coaches and match officials in the CPR training intervention would further increase the cost of the CPR intervention, regardless of whether or not they were paid for their time.

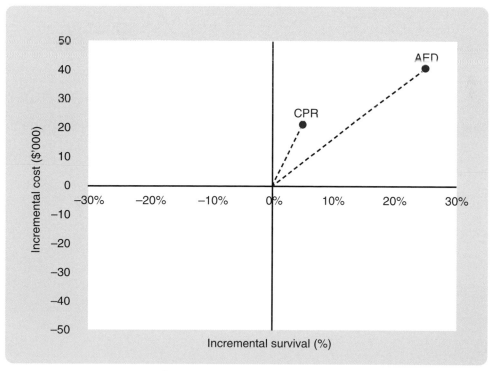

Figure 47.1 Cost-effectiveness plane

REVIEW QUESTIONS

1. When and how has cost influenced decision-making in your area of paramedicine practice or research?
2. What problems in your area of practice or research could be approached using a cost-effectiveness analysis? Try developing your own economic research questions.
3. When are cost-effectiveness analyses unlikely to provide useful information?

REFERENCES

1. Drummond M, Sculpher M, Claxton K, Stoddart G, Torrance G. Methods for the economic evaluation of health care programmes. 4th ed. Oxford, UK: Oxford University Press; 2015.
2. Aluko, P, Graybill, E, Craig, D, Henderson, C, Drummond, M, Wilson, E, et al on behalf of the Campbell and Cochrane Economics Methods Group. Chapter 20: Economic evidence. In: Higgins J, Thomas J, Chandler J, Cumpston M, Li T, Page M, et al, editors. Cochrane Handbook for Systematic Reviews of Interventions version 6.1. Cochrane; 2020.
3. Mogyorosy Z, Smith P. The main methodological issues in costing health care services: a literature review. Research Paper No.7. York, UK: Centre for Health Economics; 2005.
4. Foo J, Cook D, Tolsgaard M, Rivers G, Cleland J, Walsh K, et al. How to conduct cost and value analyses in health professions education: AMEE Guide No. 139. Medical Teacher. 2020;43(9):984–98.
5. Ramsey SD, Willke RJ, Glick H, Reed SD, Augustovski F, Jonsson B, et al. Cost-effectiveness analysis alongside clinical trials II—an ISPOR Good Research Practices Task Force report. Value in Health. 2015 Mar 1;18(2):161–72.
6. Baker R, Ruting B. Environmental policy analysis: a guide to non-market valuation. Canberra: Productivity Commission; 2014.
7. Sanders G, Neumann P, Basu A, Brock D, Feeny D, Krahn M, et al. Recommendations for conduct, methodological practices, and reporting of cost-effectiveness analyses: Second Panel on Cost-Effectiveness in Health and Medicine. JAMA. 2016;316(10):1093–103.
8. Husereau D, Drummond M, Petrou S, Carswell C, Moher D, Greenberg D, et al. Consolidated health economic evaluation reporting standards (CHEERS)—explanation and elaboration: a report of the ISPOR health economic evaluation publication guidelines good reporting practices task force. Value Health. 2013;16(2):231–50.

Sharing New Knowledge

Previous sections of this textbook have provided the reader with a broad insight into the varied world of research. Section 1 introduced the reader to the idea of research, provided suggestions on where to begin and stressed why it is important that research in the area of paramedicine continues to grow and evolve. Section 2 focused on the crucial aspect of preparation, both by understanding and evaluating what others have done before us, as well as thinking about challenges like sampling and bias, that can have significant effects on our research outcomes. Section 3 presented key aspects of quantitative research, looking at research designs and analysis approaches that can help answer research hypothesis, using numbers and statistical methods. Section 4 described qualitative research methodologies and gave insights into methods and analysis to provide a more person-centred investigation as to why we may see the outcomes that we do. And finally, Section 5 outlined other research approaches that give researchers different methodologies to answer varied questions.

The aim of all the previous sections was to introduce the reader to the extremely varied world of research, and to arm them with the foundation skills necessary to start their research project. The challenge from here is to make sure your research is available to others, and that is the aim of this coming section.

By sending your work to a journal or a conference committee, you open up your work to peer review, which is vital in research. Peer review asks experienced researchers, who are not linked to your project, to read your work for rigour and validity. More often than not, this only increases the quality of your work. Presenting your work (in any format) also allows others to learn from your outcomes, which can lead to changes in the way they care for their patients and themselves. Either way, although sharing your knowledge may not be the first thing you think about when you start research, it is perhaps the most important step to making your findings, no matter how big or small, contribute to the future of paramedicine.

48

Writing and Getting Your Research Published

Brett Williams and Peter O'Meara

LEARNING OUTCOMES

1. Understand the importance of publishing research
2. Recall the authorship guidelines and principles
3. Explain IMRaD: Introduction, Methods, Results and Discussion for publications
4. Describe the importance of using the Enhancing the QUAlity and Transparency Of health Research (EQUATOR) network
5. Contrast the pros and cons of publishing in traditional versus open access journals

INTRODUCTION

Getting your research published and disseminated as wide and far as possible is critical to the research process. Reasons for publishing your research may include: to change practice, allow examination of your work, educate others, pool knowledge and expertise, obtain grant funding, career advancement and promotion.[1] This might take the form of a full-text publication, full-text conference proceeding or book chapter, for example, and requires careful and a well-planned process to achieve publication of your work. Equally important is that publishing in peer-reviewed journals and books and presenting to conferences validates your research. Following a systematic process and writing 'template' can significantly help in the writing phase and having your work peer-reviewed and published to the world. This chapter outlines five phases ensuring a systematic writing and publishing process.

PHASE 1: PRE-WRITING

First, be clear: what do you have to say? What is important to say about your research and what does the supporting or conflicting literature say about your work and its findings? Other things to consider early on are what is the right format for your work, what is the audience (best authorship impact) for your work and where should you publish your work and findings.

Authorship

To avoid potentially awkward conversations, have this conversation very early with your co-authors and make it clear what writing expectations and timeframes are required; make sure this is documented too. Make sure any conflicts of interest are also addressed at this stage. Generally, and broadly, authorship is based on a substantial contribution to: the conception design; acquisition of data; analysis and interpretation of data; drafting of the article or revising it

BOX 48.1 ICMJE Authoring Criteria

The ICMJE recommends that authorship be based on the following four criteria:

1. substantial contributions to the conception or design of the work; or the acquisition, analysis or interpretation of data for the work AND
2. drafting the work or revising it critically for important intellectual content AND
3. final approval of the version to be published AND
4. agreement to be accountable for all aspects of the work in ensuring that questions related to the accuracy or integrity of any part of the work are appropriately investigated and resolved.

In addition to being accountable for the parts of the work he or she has done, an author should be able to identify which co-authors are responsible for specific other parts of the work. In addition, authors should have confidence in the integrity of the contributions of their co-authors.

All those designated as authors should meet all four criteria for authorship, and all who meet the four criteria should be identified as authors. Those who do not meet all four criteria should be acknowledged.

Source: International Committee of Medical Journal Editors (ICMJE). Defining the role of authors and contributors. 2022. Online. Available: https://www.icmje.org/recommendations/browse/roles-and-responsibilities/defining-the-role-of-authors-and-contributors.html.

and approving the final version to be published. Multiple ethical authorship guidelines exist and are applied by journals accordingly. A very common authorship guideline is the International Committee of Medical Journal Editors (ICMJE) at https://www.icmje.org/recommendations/browse/roles-and-responsibilities/defining-the-role-of-authors-and-contributors.html. See Box 48.1.

Another good resource to review is the guidelines on good publication practice from the Committee on Publication Ethics (COPE) at https://publicationethics.org/.

PHASE 2: WRITING

This is the most difficult and time-consuming part. Some writing tips include making it a regular activity, losing the imposter syndrome and 'what if it's not good enough' thoughts, setting clear and achievable goals, mind mapping and getting some feedback. Your writing style is important to also consider, particularly when you are first starting your publishing career. Make sure to leave clear 'signposts'

for the readers and that your paragraphs with major and minor arguments are coherent, logical and clearly linked. Structure is everything.

While each journal will have its own author writing guidelines, the structure and basics of writing a paper should remain consistent. A common mnemonic is IMRaD (Introduction, Methods, Results and Discussion) and should be your writing template (see the following sections). Also, carefully consider a concise yet catchy title if you can and please make sure you use appropriate MeSH terms in your keywords. You can find these through the National Library of Medicine at https://www.ncbi.nlm.nih.gov/mesh.

Introduction: Why Did You Do It?

The introduction provides background to the article. Search the literature to find out what is known about the topic, whether others have done similar work and if they have, whether their work was sound, robust and generalisable. This should then lead to why there is a gap, and why this gap is important to address and answer. Remember, your detailed discussion of previous literature belongs in the discussion and not the introduction (this is a common error). The last sentence of your introduction should succinctly and accurately describe what you aimed to find out in the study.

Methods: What Did You Do?

This section is very structured and should contain sections such as design, population, sampling technique, procedures, intervention (if used), instrumentation, data analysis (quantitative, qualitative or mixed methods), trial numbers and ethical considerations. For informed readers, this is the most important section. An excellent and very important resource is the Equator Network: Enhancing the QUAlity and Transparency Of health Research (EQUATOR) at https://www.equator-network.org/. This site includes multiple reporting guidelines (i.e. cross-sectional studies, randomised studies, systematic reviews, mixed methods, Delphi studies) in an attempt to improve the reliability and trustworthiness of published health research literature. Note: Do not retrospectively use these guidelines; these should be used before any data collection is undertaken.

Results: What Did You Find?

Stick to what is relevant and adds to the research aim and research question(s). It is often useful to 'signpost' the research questions in this section, making it explicitly clear to the reader what data is being presented, why and which part of the study results are being presented. Be sure to include basic descriptive and participative data. The text should tell the story, while tables give the evidence and figures illustrate the highlights. This is important to help avoid repetition of information.

Discussion: What Might It Mean?

Start with a summary of the main findings and the meaning of the study. What are the possible mechanisms and implications for clinicians or policymakers? Compare and contrast your findings with a critical review of previous similar research. Ensure clear descriptions of the strengths and weaknesses of the study in relation to other studies. Why might we have got different results? What might the study mean? What questions remain unanswered and what is the next step?

You will also need to include an abstract (again, often in IMRaD format), limitations and future research section, conclusion, references, acknowledgments and usually a conflict of interest statement. Again, follow the journal's authorship style guides.

PHASE 3: PUBLISHING

Now to the good part—but be warned that other associated work will still be needed as well as time. Publishing is generally not a quick process. Before you submit your work, consider asking a colleague who is not involved in the research to read your paper. Ask them to give you feedback on whether it is easy to read, easy to understand, free of hyperbole and contains clear aims and arguments. Also ask them if there are obvious typographical or grammatical errors and whether the paper itself is interesting (does it addresses the 'so what' question; see Phase 4).

Whatever type of research you are publishing, it is important that you avoid any suggestion of plagiarism, which is defined as the use of other peoples' ideas or words without acknowledging the source. Similar principles apply to self-plagiarism, which is either reusing your already-published work without acknowledgment or alternately recycling data that you have already reported in another form. Journals and reviewers will pick up plagiarism either through specific detection software or their own experience and expertise.

Picking the most appropriate journal to publish in can be quite difficult depending on the topic. Fortunately, there are resources to help with this, such as Journal Author Name Estimator (JANE) (http://jane.biosemantics.org/). Be familiar with journal metrics and academic metrics (if applicable) as well as journal impact versus readership impact. It is also important to be clear about what types of articles the journal accepts or not, and whether you wish to publish in a traditional journal versus open access. Be wary of some open access journals as they may be predatory in nature; check using Cabell's Predatory Reports at

https://www2.cabells.com/about-predatory. Think. Check. Submit. at https://thinkchecksubmit.org/ is another good resource to help with publishing your work.

PHASE 4: PEER-REVIEW

Make sure you are patient at this stage and are prepared for criticism. What do editors/reviewers look for? The first thing is the 'so what' question; that is, is the paper of genuine interest, reads well and makes sense, and will add enough to existing knowledge? If the paper does not fit the journal's general aims and scope, it will likely be rejected at the editorial phase and not sent out for peer review.

Ensure you have read and followed the journal's style guide carefully; if you haven't, the paper will be sent back to address and fix the issues, wasting time. If your paper is sent out for peer review, expect reviews to range from accepting with minor or major changes to outright rejection. These reviews usually take 2 to 3 months to be returned. If your paper is accepted pending changes made based on suggestions by the peer reviewers, then some general principles need to be followed. Read the reviewer's comments and then read them again. Do the reviewers have a point? Try not to be too defensive. Think about how you can improve your paper based on their comments. If you disagree or they are wrong, then you do not need to make direct changes to the paper; however, you will need to justify why changes have not been made. Do not be rude in your responses.

PHASE 5: POST-PUBLICATION AND DISSEMINATION

The final and most exciting stage is post-publication and dissemination. At this stage, it is important to have some form of dissemination strategy in place. Your publication must reach the right and most important audiences, particularly those without university library access or access to journal articles. Use of social media and other web-based platforms for dissemination is vital, and tracking the data/influence of your work (altmetrics) is equally important. Signing up to sites such as Research Gate, Publons and Academia allows you to promote your work and make new connections with other like-minded researchers, and may lead to potential collaborators. Presenting your work at conferences is another important dissemination strategy. Dissemination is discussed in more detail in Chapter 49.

CONCLUSION

Having your research published and disseminated widely is vital to the development of knowledge and science. Time, effort and well-planned project management skills are all required in getting your research published. This chapter has outlined five phases to ensure you use a systematic process and writing 'template' that should help significantly in publishing your work in peer-reviewed literature.

REVIEW QUESTIONS

1. You are about to start a research project and the issue of authorship has not been discussed. Which resources and guidelines would you use to initiate a discussion about authorship?
2. Are there issues with publishing your research from higher degree by research (i.e. a master degree, a PhD)? If so, why or why not?
3. Why is it important to use 'official' MeSH terms in your published research?
4. What are the ethical issues surrounding publishing in open access journals (not predatory) that charge researchers thousands of dollars to publish?
5. You have received an email from an unknown journal you suspect might be a predatory publication. On what basis would you determine whether you should consider submitting your work to this journal?
6. What copyright issues should you consider before presenting your form from a publication at a peer-reviewed conference?

SUGGESTED FURTHER READING

Grudniewicz A, Moher D, Cobey KD, Bryson GL, Cukier S, Allen K, et al. Predatory journals: no definition, no defence. Nature. 2019; 576:210-12. Online. Available: https://www.nature.com/articles/d41586-019-03759-y.

Murray R. Writing for an academic journal: 10 tips. The Guardian. 7 September 2013. Online. Available: http://www.theguardian.com/higher-education-network/blog/2013/sep/06/academic-journal-writing-top-tips.

SCImago Journal & Country Rank: https://www.scimagojr.com/index.php.

Shaikh AA. 7 steps to publishing in a scientific journal. Elsevier Connect. 4 April 2016. Online. Available: https://www.elsevier.com/connect/7-steps-to-publishing-in-a-scientific-journal.

The Conversation: http://theconversation.com/au

Web of Science: http://mjl.clarivate.com/home

REFERENCE

1. Thistlethwaite J, Anderson E. Writing for publication: increasing the likelihood of success. Journal of Interprofessional Care. 2021;35(5):784-90.

49

Research Dissemination and Bibliometrics

Bronwyn Beovich

LEARNING OUTCOMES

1. To gain an understanding of the importance of research dissemination and the methods that may be utilised to facilitate dissemination

2. To understand the concept of bibliometrics and their use in quantification of the characteristics of a body of literature

DEFINITION

- Research dissemination: The sharing of research findings to targeted audiences to enable the information to be utilised.[1] This information should be accessible and understandable, and can be used in decision-making and applied in practice if relevant. It is a vital step in the process of knowledge translation and integration into evidence-based practice.[1]
- Bibliometrics: Involves the quantitative analysis of a body of literature with regards to features such as publishing journal, author characteristics and citation number.[2]

INTRODUCTION

As the previous chapter suggested, dissemination or communication of research findings to relevant audiences should be considered an essential component of the research process and is a fundamental responsibility of researchers.[3] It enables development in cognate areas, facilitates collaboration between researchers and other stakeholders, and enhances community engagement.[4] Without dissemination, research output cannot be transferred into clinical knowledge or best-practice guidelines or contribute to evidence-based practice.[5–7]

Research dissemination may take many forms, with traditional avenues including peer-reviewed journal articles, conference presentations/papers, workshops, seminars and books/book chapters.[3] However, internet capabilities have opened up many relatively innovative modalities that may be utilised for rapid communication of research to a worldwide audience. For example, social media (e.g. Twitter, Instagram, Facebook), podcasts, websites, as well as other online formats such as LinkedIn, ResearchGate, Academia.edu and YouTube (e.g. TED talks) can all be used for this purpose.

The extent of dissemination and impact of research output may be quantitively examined via bibliometric analysis,[8] with the conventional unit of measurement being the citation count. That is, the number of times a research paper has been cited by, and is therefore influential to, other research. Although citation count has inherent limitations, it is one of the most widely used methods for judging the impact of research findings.[9] The value of this approach is based on the notion that more important papers are more likely to be cited and thus the citation count is a direct measure of recognition and impact on a particular field of research.[10] It can be used to measure the research impact of a researcher, research department, university, professional discipline, country, as well as providing information on collaboration and emerging research topics.

Bibliometric information may be accessed via many databases; all of which possess different characteristics and capabilities. Even the established academic databases of Web of Science, Scopus and Google Scholar have diversity with regards to various operational features. These include date and subject coverage, number of records, journal inclusion, specificity and ease of use. The choice of database(s) to use should be decided with consideration of factors such as the magnitude of coverage for the relevant research area and the particular information required.[11]

There are multiple journal-level citation metrics in common use (see Table 49.1), all with advantages, disadvantages and limitations which need to be considered.

Metrics are also available at an article level (e.g. PlumX) and author level (e.g. h-index).

- PlumX captures traditional citation metrics along with metrics primarily associated with social media such as 'clicks', 'likes' and 'tweets'.
- The h-index is formulated on the basis that an author has 'h' number of publications that have been cited at least 'h' times. It is a measure of an author's productivity and impact.

Authors are able to set up an account to track their citation metrics. For example, within Google Scholar you can create a profile (which can be public or private). Information on articles which you have authored will then be available and your h-index will be provided. You can click 'Follow' to create an alert that lets you know when someone cites one of your publications.

The continued adoption of social media within academia has necessitated the development of new metrics with the ability to consider information circulated online. The term 'altmetrics' signifies alternative metrics, and are data that can provide information indicative of the dissemination and impact of online information.[12] It measures online attention in the form of entities such as tweets, likes, comments, shares, views, tags and downloads. Although altmetric data can be rapidly generated, have broad and diverse coverage, and are freely available, there are inherent limitations such as heterogeneity of measurements and in extent of peer review.[13]

The correlation between traditional research metrics and altmetrics has not been fully elucidated, with correlations between the two ranging from strongly positive[14] to low or negligible[10]. This suggests that the information captured by each approach may be fundamentally different. Therefore, metrics derived from social media sources should not be viewed as a substitute to traditional citation analysis, but perhaps a valuable adjunct.

TABLE 49.1 Journal-Level Citation Metrics in Common Use

Metric	Database Utilised (Organisation)	Method of Determination and Information
Journal impact factor (IF)	Web of Science (Clarivate)	Calculated by dividing the number of citations in the Journal Citation Reports (JCR) year by the total number of citable items published in the previous two years.
Eigenfactor® score (ES)	Web of Science (Clarivate)	Measures the number of times articles from a journal published in the past 5 years have been cited in the JCR year. References from one article in a journal to another article from the same journal are removed, so that ES is not influenced by journal self-citation.
Article Influence™ Score (AIS)	Web of Science (Clarivate)	This is calculated by dividing the journal's ES by the number of articles published by the journal, normalised as a fraction of all articles in all publications. It measures the relative importance of the journal on a per-article basis, while considering the size of the journal.
CiteScore	Scopus (Elsevier)	CiteScore is the average of the sum of the citations received in a given year to publications published in the previous 3 years, divided by the sum of publications in the same 3 years.
SCImago journal rank (SJR)	Scopus (Elsevier)	Citations are weighted with regard to the publishing journal over a period of 3 years. A citation's value is greater for those within high-SCR journals compared with those from a low-SCR journal.
Source-Normalised Impact per Paper (SNIP)	Scopus (Elsevier)	Citations are weighted with regard to the citation numbers within a particular subject over a period of 3 years. A citation's value is greater for journals in fields where citations are less likely, thus enabling comparison of journals from different fields.

Sources: Clarivate. Web of Science and related products. 2022. Online. Available: https://support.clarivate.com/Scientificand AcademicResearch. Elsevier. Measuring a journal's impact. 2022. Online. Available: https://www.elsevier.com/authors/tools-and-resources/measuring-a-journals-impact. SCImago Journal & Country Rank. Online. Available: https://www.scimagojr.com/.

CONCLUSION

The dissemination of research findings is an integral component of the research process, as information can only be useful if it is efficiently communicated to relevant audiences. Although many metrics are available to measure engagement with and impact of research, all tools have inherent strengths and weaknesses which need to be considered in the selection of a method for literature examination. The use of a combination of bibliometric methods may be a reasonable approach to enable the capture of information from diverse sources of research engagement and impact.

REVIEW QUESTIONS

1. At what point in the research process should planning the dissemination of research output take place?
2. With the increasing use of social media, will there always be a place for traditional citation-based bibliometrics?

SUGGESTED FURTHER READING

Beovich B, Olaussen A, Williams B. A bibliometric analysis of paramedicine publications: 2010–2019. (Under review)

Olaussen A, Beovich B, Williams B. Top 100 cited paramedicine papers: A bibliometric study. Emergency Medicine Australasia. 2021. Online. Available: https://doi.org/10.1111/1742-6723.13774.

Roldan-Valadez E, Salazar-Ruiz SY, Ibarra-Contreras R, Rios C. Current concepts on bibliometrics: a brief review about impact factor, Eigenfactor score, CiteScore, SCImago journal rank, source-normalised impact per paper, h-index, and alternative metrics. Irish Journal of Medical Science (1971–). 2019;188(3):939–51.

REFERENCES

1. National Institute for Health Research. How to disseminate your research. 2019. Online. Available: https://www.nihr.ac.uk/documents/how-to-disseminate-your-research/19951.
2. van Raan A. Measuring science: basic principles and application of advanced bibliometrics. In: Glänzel W, Moed HF, Schmoch U, Thelwall M, editors. Springer Handbook of Science and Technology Indicators. Cham: Springer International Publishing. 2019;237–80.
3. Marín-González E, Malmusi D, Camprubí L, Borrell C. The role of dissemination as a fundamental part of a research project: lessons learned from SOPHIE. International Journal of Health Services. 2017;47(2):258–76.
4. National Health and Medical Research Council. Dissemination and communication. 2019. Online. Available: https://www.nhmrc.gov.au/guidelinesforguidelines/implement/dissemination-and-communication#_ENREF_1.
5. Edwards DJ. Dissemination of research results: on the path to practice change. The Canadian Journal of Hospital Pharmacy. 2015;68(6):465.
6. Neta G, Glasgow RE, Carpenter CR, Grimshaw JM, Rabin BA, Fernandez ME, et al. A framework for enhancing the value of research for dissemination and implementation. American Journal of Public Health. 2015;105(1):49–57.
7. Milat AJ, Bauman AE, Redman S, Curac N. Public health research outputs from efficacy to dissemination: a bibliometric analysis. BMC Public Health. 2011;11(1):1–9.
8. Thompson DF, Walker CK. A descriptive and historical review of bibliometrics with applications to medical sciences. Pharmacotherapy: The Journal of Human Pharmacology and Drug Therapy. 2015;35(6):551–9.
9. Kratz JE, Strasser C. Making data count. Scientific Data. 2015;2(1):1–5.
10. Barbic D, Tubman M, Lam H, Barbic S. An analysis of altmetrics in emergency medicine. Academic Emergency Medicine. 2016;23(3):251–68.
11. Moral-Muñoz JA, Herrera-Viedma E, Santisteban-Espejo A, Cobo MJ. Software tools for conducting bibliometric analysis in science: an up-to-date review. El Profesional de la Información. 2020;29(1):e290103.
12. Altmetric. Sources of attention. 2021. Online. Available: https://www.altmetric.com/about-our-data/our-sources/.
13. Fang Z, Costas R, Tian W, Wang X, Wouters P. An extensive analysis of the presence of altmetric data for Web of Science publications across subject fields and research topics. Scientometrics. 2020;124(3):2519–49.
14. Ouchi A, Saberi MK, Ansari N, Hashempour L, Isfandyari-Moghaddam A. Do altmetrics correlate with citations? A study based on the 1,000 most-cited articles. Information Discovery and Delivery. 2019;47(4):192–202.

50

The Implementation (Translation) Process

Leon Baranowski

LEARNING OUTCOMES

1. Develop an understanding of knowledge translation
2. Identify types of knowledge translation
3. Implementation of action cycles and process

DEFINITION

The implementation process can be defined as the exchange, synthesis and ethically sound application of knowledge within a complex system to accelerate the capture of the benefits of research for improved health, more-effective services and products and a strengthened healthcare system.[1]

INTRODUCTION

Many terms have been used to describe the process of putting knowledge into action.[2] These include knowledge creation (primary research), knowledge distillation (the creation of systematic reviews and guidelines) and knowledge dissemination (appearances in journals and presentations). These aspects of knowledge translation are not enough on their own to ensure the utilisation of new knowledge in paramedic decision-making.[3] Many proposed theories and frameworks exist for the practice of knowledge translation, which can be confusing in practice.[4] A conceptual framework developed by Graham and colleagues, termed the knowledge-to-action cycle, provides an approach that builds on the commonalities found in a review of planned action theories.[2]

It's important to remember that the process of translating knowledge to action is an iterative, dynamic and complex process. It concerns the creation and application (action cycle) of knowledge. Although it is drawn as a cycle, those using it may need to use the phases out of sequence, depending on the project or practice to implement. When using this

process, it is essential that the paramedics and any other users of the knowledge are included to ensure that the knowledge and its subsequent implementation are relevant to their needs. The funnel of knowledge creation and the major action steps or stages comprising the model for translating knowledge to action are illustrated in Figure 50.1.[5]

EXAMPLES

It's important to consider the size of the knowledge translation you are looking to implement. Some examples of the types of changes may lend themselves to different internal processes based on your available platforms. As organisations embrace the digital age with app solutions, there are more options to affect change more dynamically.[6]

Examples of research that can affect organisations could come in the areas of practice shown in Table 50.1.

An example could be a small-scale practice update and guideline release. It could be as something as simple as a medication dosage change, new medication or change in the way we support palliative care patients which you are looking to translate into practice. As we do this, we need to consider our end users and how we progress through the cycle. Who are the users? What is the level of education/clinical role? Can this be something that we communicate through our apps and guidelines, or with written communication? Or do we need a session with an educator? Maybe it's both! Could we deliver this at a local level with some follow-up using audits? Or are we better positioning this as a wider update with more of a formal sign off? Once you are satisfied that you have addressed questions similar to

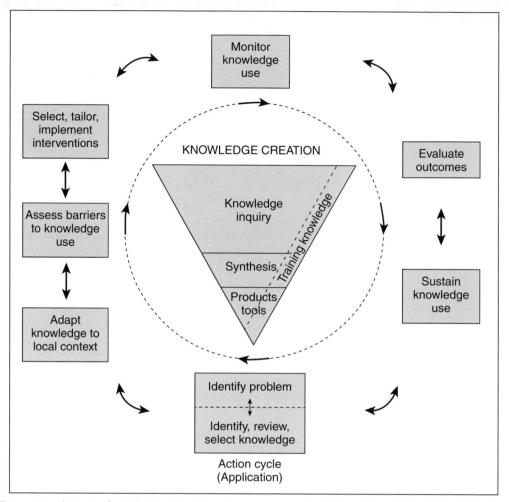

Figure 50.1 Journey of continuing education (Source: Graham I, Logan J, Harrison M, Straus S, Tetroe J, Caswell W, Robinson N. Lost in knowledge translation: time for a map? Journal of Continuing Education in the Health Professions. 2006;26(1):13–24. Online. Available: https://doi.org/10.1002/chp.47.)

TABLE 50.1	Examples of Paramedic Practice Areas and Change
Paramedic Practice	**System and Organisational Changes**
Small-scale practice updates	Education
Guidelines and protocols	Models of care
Equipment and medications	Service delivery
Assessments	Pathways
Quality, key performance indicators and care bundles	Clinical governance

this, you will be able to decide on the approach that is right for your organisation and the correct process.

Successful implementation usually requires an active change process aimed to achieve both individual- and organisational-level uses. Individuals may actively promote the implementation process and could come from the inner or outer setting (e.g. local champions, external change agents). The implementation process may develop into an interrelated series of subprocesses that do not necessarily occur sequentially. In this situation, perhaps you may need to make your leaders and educators aware before the rest of the workforce so they can be prepared and armed with the evidence to support any questions. There are often related processes progressing simultaneously at multiple levels within the organisation.[7] These subprocesses may be formally planned or spontaneous, conscious or subconscious, linear or nonlinear; but ideally they are all aimed in the same general direction: effective implementation.[6]

Knowledge translation is as much about understanding the climate and opportunities within your own organisation for advancing practice, as it is about change management. Knowledge translation can be thought of as the transfer of knowledge from research into clinical practice, but it is ultimately about capturing and disseminating information to ensure its application.[8]

Efficiency in the uptake of evidence-based research is essential in paramedic practice, as it is with other healthcare professions. It's important that evidence-based research is efficiently translated into paramedic practice as such strategies serve to improve patient outcomes and reduce system inefficiencies, thereby strengthening out-of-hospital care and the broader continuum of healthcare.[9]

CONCLUSION

With the rise of academic paramedics and the growing body of literature created by paramedics, knowledge translation will continue to be an integral part of organisational change and developments as we continue to explore and refine how we can improve the care we provide to patients. Ambulance services and large health organisations must ensure that research and development is supported and continues to grow as well as remain a core part of an organisation's strategy.

REVIEW QUESTIONS

1. You have been asked to implement a medication dosage change to a clinical practice guideline which is used as a basic standard of care for your organisation. What approach would you take to this change? Which parts of the action cycle would you use?
2. A new piece of evidence has been released and published by a national organisation in best practice for trauma care. How would you evaluate the research and application of the knowledge and practice to your system? What impacts would this have, and how would you implement the change?

REFERENCES

1. Canadian Institutes of Health Research. Knowledge Translation Strategy 2004-2009. Ottawa, Canada. 2004. Online. Available: https://cihr-irsc.gc.ca/e/26574.html#defining.
2. Graham I, Logan J, Harrison M, Straus S, Tetroe J, Caswell W, Robinson N. Lost in knowledge translation: time for a map? Journal of Continuing Education in the Health Professions. 2006;26(1):13–24. Online. Available: https://doi.org/10.1002/chp.47
3. Straus S, Tetroe J, Graham I. Defining knowledge translation. Canadian Medical Association Journal. 2009;181(3–4):165–8. Online. Available: https://doi.org/10.1503/cmaj.081229.
4. Graham I, Tetroe J. Some theoretical underpinnings of knowledge translation. Academic Emergency Medicine. 2007;14(11):936–41. Online. Available: https://pubmed.ncbi.nlm.nih.gov/17967955/.
5. Madon T, Hofman K, Kupfer L, Glass R. Public health: implementation science. Science. 2007:318(5857):1728–9. Online. Available: https://doi.org/10.1126/science.1150009.
6. Damschroder L, Aron D, Keith R, Kirsh S, Alexander J, Lowery J. Fostering implementation of health services research findings into practice: a consolidated framework for advancing implementation science. Implementation Science. 2009;4(1). Online. Available: https://doi.org/10.1186/1748-5908-4-50.
7. Pettigrew A, Woodman R, Cameron K. Studying organizational change and development: challenges for future research. Academy of Management Journal. 2001:44(4): 697–713. Online. Available: https://doi.org/10.5465/3069411.
8. Williams B, Jennings P, Fielder C, Ghirardello A. Next generation paramedics, agents of change, or time for curricula renewal? Advances in Medical Education And Practice. 2013:245. Online. Available: https://doi.org/10.2147/amep.s53085.
9. Straus S, Tetroe J, Graham I. Knowledge translation is the use of knowledge in health care decision making. Journal of Clinical Epidemiology. 2011:64(1):6–10. Online. Available: https://pubmed.ncbi.nlm.nih.gov/19926445/.

51

Grant Writing and Team Building

David Reid

LEARNING OUTCOMES

1. Understand the skills required to build a research team
2. Outline the research grant writing process
3. Describe the contents of a research grant
4. Source research grants

INTRODUCTION

Prior to securing a grant, the research team needs to be built. Multidisciplinary research teams have been shown to improve overall research quality when they contain both subject matter experts and research experts. In an increasingly fiscally tight research environment, good grant writing, targeted from the most appropriate funding body is essential to the paramedic researcher. This chapter outlines the key components of building a research team and writing a successful research grant.

BUILDING A RESEARCH TEAM

Increasingly across healthcare, research is being conducted in a multidisciplinary holistic environment.[1,2] Paramedicine research is no different and prehospital and unscheduled care research comprises participants from across the health and research specialties. The literature identifies three types of team formats, as shown in Figure 51.1.[3]

The benefits of multidisciplinary team research are becoming increasingly well known, in particular for research that is not randomised in nature or that has a significant qualitative element. There are many examples of paramedicine research that adopt a mixed methods approach, and a multidisciplinary research team maximises the opportunities to present legitimate and valid findings and recommendations.[1]

It has been suggested that there are three dimensions relevant to undertaking multidisciplinary team research:[4]

1. the number of people doing the research
2. the kind of actions involved in the research process
3. the number of disciplines involved in the research.

Each element is relevant to building the paramedicine research team. The research team needs to be sufficiently resourced so that all the required research tasks are achieved, yet not so big that competing interests take over. The team needs to include individuals with the relevant skills to undertake the research tasks, such as qualitative or quantitative data collection, analysis and report writing. The number of disciplines in the research team needs to reflect the environment in which the research is occurring. For instance, if the research is investigating the continuum of care from prehospital to hospital, the team should include researchers from all included clinical areas.

Diverse teams, with members from different fields, bring different mindsets and perspectives to the research being conducted. This reduces the likelihood of 'group think', which occurs when people of a common background come together and think along the same lines. As mentioned in Section 1 of this book, diverse teams also allow potential barriers to be addressed prior to the research commencing, as each person can identify issues and provide solutions relevant to their setting.

Teamwork, or the integration of individual members towards achievement of a shared goal, can be viewed though a model of effectiveness including inputs (such as team member characteristics and organisational characteristics) and outputs that depend on the effectiveness of team processes.[5] To maximise team effectiveness, Gibert

> Multidisciplinary teams
>
> • The different professions work to individually set goals and meet to discuss their progress.
>
> Interdisciplinary teams
>
> • Goals are first agreed by the team, whose members then coordinate their input to the common treatment plan.
>
> Transdisciplinary teams
>
> • Not only goals but skills are shared.

Figure 51.1 Team formats (Source: Young CA. Building a care and research team. Journal of the Neurological Sciences. 1998;160:S137–40.)

and colleagues identify a range of skills required in a research team.[6] These include research skills in qualitative or quantitative methods, as well as soft skills such as team-working, strategic thinking and initiative.

Management of the multidisciplinary research team is the responsibility of the lead researcher. Therefore, the lead researcher needs to have research and management skills. It has been hypothesised that although collaboration is common, true coordination is rare in multidisciplinary team research.[2]

Core competencies for team leaders include motivation, moderation and mentorship. The team leader needs to have the ability to connect disparate team members, especially where teams are spread geographically. A true team leader needs to be able to bring the team together during its formation stage, sustain the team during the core data collection and analysis phases and the report-writing phase.

RESEARCH GRANTS

In order to successfully undertake research, funding is required from either the researcher's own organisation or from an external funding body such as the National Health and Medical Research Council (NHMRC) in Australia, the National Science Foundation in the United States or the UK Research and Innovation Agency in the United Kingdom.

An application will almost always need to be made to a funding organisation to successfully receive grant funding. These applications are usually competitive in nature, and often more applications are received than there is money available. For this reason, a grant application needs to be of high quality in order to receive funding. As shown in Figure 51.2, the grant process starts with your research idea and ends with final publication and reporting.

A number of key principles should be considered when seeking funding for a research project.
1. Match the funding body to your project. Ensure you select a funding body which fits your idea, rather than finding a grant and seeking to fit your project to it.
2. Ensure you allocate time. Grants take time to write, so it is essential you allocate sufficient time to write a high-quality proposal.
3. Ensure that your research team is aware of the funding application and their role in the research. Where possible, involve early and mid-career researchers to build outputs and facilitate individual development.

Funding applications often have similar information required. Information commonly required on a grant application includes the following:
- overview of your organisation
- project title
- importance/significance of the research
- team composition including involvement of appropriate subject matter and/or research methodology experts
- project methodology and research approach
- timeframe
- budget (including direct financial contributions and in-kind contributions)
- anticipated outcomes and outputs
- measures of success (evaluation)
- evidence of ethics submission and/or approval
- research team and their collective and individual experience
- past grants and outputs.

Grant applications will be assessed against the funding body's criteria, usually by a funding committee. The review committee may or may not have expertise in your research

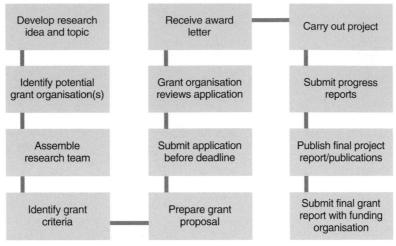

Figure 51.2 the grant process

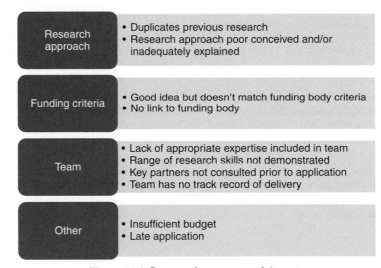

Figure 51.3 Reasons for unsuccessful grants

area; therefore, it is important that your grant application is written in plain English, for a non-technical audience. Unsuccessful grants often show common themes, as shown in Figure 51.3.[7] You may or may not receive feedback on why your grant application was unsuccessful.

CONCLUSION

Research is increasingly being conducted in multidisciplinary teams. The benefits of multidisciplinary research are well known, and the mixed methods approach is an accepted method that maximises the opportunities to present findings and recommendations which are legitimate and valid. When building a research team, sufficient resources need to be allocated, individuals need to have appropriate skills and the team needs to reflect the environment in which the research is taking place. Once the team is built, leadership is essential to maximise the research outcomes and outputs.

Grants are an essential component of research. The grant writing process should be treated as a project and, because grants are competitive in nature, sufficient time and resources need to be allocated to writing the grant. When considering a grant, you need to match the grant to your research idea, and ensure that you answer all the components of the grant application. Ensure that your grant is written in plain English and that you avoid the common errors in grant writing.

REVIEW QUESTIONS

1. When building your research teams, what are some key features you should prioritise?
2. What do diverse teams reduce the likelihood of during the research?
3. What is meant by empowering others as part of a research team?
4. Why is it important that grant applications be written in plain English?

SUGGESTED FURTHER READING

Australian Research Council: https://www.arc.gov.au/
Australian Rotary Health: https://australianrotaryhealth.org.au/research/
Grant Connect: https://www.grants.gov.au/Go/List
National Health and Medical Research Council: https://www.nhmrc.gov.au/
Research Data Australia: https://researchdata.edu.au/grants
Research Professional: http://researchprofessional.com
State health departments such as the Government of Western Australia's Department of Health: https://ww2.health.wa.gov.au/Articles/N_R/Research-funding-programs

REFERENCES

1. Saks M, Allsop J. Researching health: qualitative, quantitative and mixed methods. 3rd ed. Los Angeles: SAGE Publications; 2019.
2. Disis ML, Slattery JT. The road we must take: multidisciplinary team science. Science Translational Medicine. 2010;2(22): 22–9.
3. Young CA. Building a care and research team. Journal of the Neurological Sciences. 1998;160:S137–40.
4. Lamson RW. The present strains between science and government. Social Forces. 1954;33(4):360–7.
5. Driskell JE, Salas E, Driskell T. Foundations of teamwork and collaboration. American Psychologist. 2018;73(4):334–48.
6. Gibert A, Tozer WC, Westoby M. Teamwork, soft skills, and research training. Trends in Ecology & Evolution. 2017;32(2): 81–4.
7. Greater Victoria Community Funders Network. Grant writing handbook. Melbourne, Victoria: Greater Victoria Community Funders' Network; 2020.

52

Setting Up the Future of Paramedicine

Walter Tavares

LEARNING OUTCOMES

1. Describe three broad activities for those in the paramedicine profession to consider when thinking about the future of paramedicine

2. Describe structural ways of organising paramedicine that support a positive and successful future

INTRODUCTION

What is the future of paramedicine? Anticipating, seeking or predicting the future on most topics is, in many instances, a challenge. Indeed, forecasting the future has been described as being 'as accurate as a dart-throwing chimpanzee'—in other words, as good as random guessing.[1] Making predictions has also been described as a 'Lorentzian cloud'.[1] That is, even if one knows all that there is to know about how clouds forms, so many complex interactions mean a final form cannot be reliably predicted. Instead, we must wait and see. There are obviously limits on predictions in a complex world, but thinking about the future is not pointless. Asking such a question provides opportunities for careful and deep reflection. Articulating that reflective process can, rather than claim to reach the 'correct' vision of the future, provide the self and others stimulus to pause and reflect and be generative (i.e. lead to new ideas). Also, over time, contexts and people, generative insights become increasingly refined and more meaningful. This chapter provides ways of stimulating that process by discussing three ways of thinking about the future of paramedicine, such that the future looks different (for the better) than it does now.

A SHARED PLACE TO START

The first is a near future, and one where paramedicine is guided by a *shared conceptual framework*. These frameworks provide a collective but flexible understanding and way of seeing and thinking about paramedicine, while permitting a kind of flexibility for local contexts. For instance, a future paramedic would move past identity crises and have clarity guided by conceptual assumptions and commitments. In many jurisdictions, paramedicine emerged as (and perhaps still is) a resuscitation or stabilising and transport-based model or concept. This is changing, and has changed of course, but change is often driven first by local opportunities rather than a collective agreement about what paramedicine is. This is not to discount how natural and necessary evolutionary activities can be fruitful, but only to suggest some value in leveraging those experiences for broader understanding. As an example of a shared conceptual framework for future paramedics, and in response to a diverse network of paramedics in Canada, the Paramedic Chiefs of Canada commissioned a study to explore the future of paramedicine.[2] The aim was to generate a shared view about what paramedicine is for the near future. That work led to a set of principles that, if adopted widely, provide an opportunity for a collective way forward. Whether these are the right principles or not is not the point. Rather, it is the process and outcomes of working through the opportunities, challenges and limitations of a shared understanding that a future paramedic should have a handle on.

BEING COORDINATED IN OUR RESPONSE

The second is to organise paramedicine in a way that permits a *coordinated response* to future events, circumstances or ideas. Two contemporary examples might include the response to advances in artificial intelligence or other technologies, or social inequities. Groups are already working on both, but a future paramedic would see both more coordinated in our activities and distributed in their lessons and contributions in response to new realities or ideas. With an ever-changing world, paramedicine (i.e. the profession broadly) of the future will need to be equipped to shift and evolve quickly, nationally and internationally, and avoid what might otherwise reflect chaotic responses or activities. This will require an organised profession, a community of adequately positioned and skilled stakeholders, leaders, policy makers and scholars, and a supportive infrastructure (e.g. ways of detecting and selecting meaningful events, national or international databases, a pipeline for knowledge development). Systems will need to see value in contributing and participating in how paramedicine is or should be connected more broadly, and to participate in reciprocal high-quality exchange of meaningful events (i.e. where impact is a potentially broad issue), ideas and their solutions.

SUPPORTING MOONSHOTS

The third, which is intended to support a more distant future, is to foster an environment that supports the equivalent of 'moonshots'. These are spaces for *grand innovative ideas* rooted in sciences and innovations of all kinds and disciplines, permitting paramedicine to thrive in yet-to-be discovered or identified ways. Here, we might be less coordinated to permit creativity but coordinated in structuring an environment or context that promotes the advancement of paramedicine and its contributions to society, to healthcare or to any other area deemed suitable and appropriate. The goal would be to be 'better'—even if only incrementally—in these and other evolving areas for a greater impact on the world. It would again require the development of an infrastructure, pipeline and connection to other fields, disciplines, industries and funders, and ways of drawing those groups into paramedicine and what it can offer. A future paramedic would permit this kind of aspiration with opportunity, inspiration and speed. Fill in the blank: *What if paramedicine _____? That kind of creativity should be energised, unfettered, supported and part of our future.

CONCLUSION

While these three ideas may seem abstract, and perhaps not what one thinks of when asked about the future (e.g. I did not discuss technological advances), the implications for setting up and benefiting from such a future are practical, meaningful and exciting. When thinking about a future in paramedicine, others have described the need to depart from vocational thinking[3], to think of paramedicine as a profession[4], to promote better gender balance[5], for higher education[6], for revised regulatory frameworks[7] and to achieve numerous clinical advances[8]. Many of these ideas are already underway to different extents around the world. These all have merit and what they have in common are instances and glimpses of forward-looking thinking that are grounded in reflections and perhaps inspiration and creativity. A future paramedic would collectively value this, but also harness, elaborate and create a setting where this thinking can be expanded and used. A future of a 1. shared conceptual framework, 2. a coordinated response network and 3. an environment that promotes 'moonshots' perhaps steps back from these very clear and concrete examples. Instead, it is a future that meaningfully and productively aligns with and organises the profession, and fosters space for thinking big, such that the settings, systems and people it involves and serves can benefit. These ideas are intended to be more about settings than things, which provide opportunities for new and exciting futures, captured and stimulated at different time points, when new reflections and directions can be made. It may be in converting what may feel like abstract concepts into reality, and affording generative space—that is, setting up the future of paramedicine—that provides the most possible, accessible and impactful future for paramedicine.

REVIEW QUESTIONS

1. What might need to change for paramedic to foster the three ideas presented in this chapter?
2. What might be missing in these views when considering the future of paramedicine?
3. What immediate next step(s) can you take to put these ideas into action?

SUGGESTED FURTHER READING

Tavares W, Allana A, Beaune L, Weiss D, Blanchard, I. Principles to guide the future of paramedicine in Canada. Prehospital Emergency Care. 2021. Online. Available: http://doi.org/10.1080/10903127.2021.1965680.

REFERENCES

1. Tetlock PE, Gardner D. Superforecasting: the art and science of prediction. 2016: Random House.
2. Tavares W, Allana A, Beaune L, Weiss D, Blanchard I. Principles to guide the future of paramedicine in Canada. Prehospital Emergency Care. 2021;1–16.
3. O'Meara P. Student research: the future of paramedicine. Australasian Journal of Paramedicine. 2014;11(5).
4. Reed B, Cowin LS, O'Meara P, Wilson IG. Professionalism and professionalisation in the discipline of paramedicine. Australasian Journal of Paramedicine. 2019;16:1–10.
5. Mason PS, Delport S, Batt AM. Let's make this our 'thing'. Leveling the playing field for a brighter future in paramedicine. 2018. Faculty and Staff Publications—Public Safety;26–27
6. O'Meara PF, Furness S, Gleeson R. Educating paramedics for the future: a holistic approach. Journal of Health and Human Services Administration, 2017;219–53.
7. Acker JJ. Informing our future: the development of a regulatory framework for registered paramedics in Australia. Australasian Journal of Paramedicine. 2016;13(2).
8. Olaussen A, Beovich B, Williams B. Top 100 cited paramedicine papers: a bibliometric study. Emergency Medicine Australasia. April 2021;33(6).

53

Summary, Recommendations and Conclusions

Alexander Olaussen, Kelly-Ann Bowles, Bill Lord and Brett Williams

As has been highlighted in this book, paramedicine as a profession is well established in many countries and rapidly emerging in others. Research is an integral component of any profession as a means of generating knowledge to inform practice, and we are pleased to have been able to put together a research text dedicated to paramedics and those studying within paramedicine. Underpinning a profession is an establishment of a unique body of knowledge, and we hope that having engaged with this text has developed your interest in research and that your knowledge of research methods leads you to opportunities to contribute to the field. We hope that this book, with its real-life out-of-hospital and paramedic-related examples, serves your learning needs.

Paramedicine is about people, networks and collaboration. That is why we are very thankful to the many contributing authors from the four corners of the globe. In Section 1 of the book, we introduced you to research from a historical and professional perspective. In Section 2 we described how to prepare for research, followed by Section 3's discussion of how to conduct quantitative research. Section 4 described the practices of qualitative research, while Section 5 described other methodologies. Lastly, Section 6 discussed writing and the importance of disseminating and implementing research outcomes. By having many short and succinct chapters throughout, we trust the textbook will serve as a quick-reference guide as well as a complete overall and broad curriculum.

Our final recommendation, beyond the hundreds delivered throughout the book, is simply to get involved with research. It is the experience of the editors (and we are certain we speak for most of the authors) that the challenges and frustrations that may be felt   particularly early in one's research career—dawn in comparison to the positive feelings of collaboration, contribution to the profession and helping 'more than one patient' at a time. As the saying goes, give me six hours to chop down a tree and I will spend the first four sharpening the axe. We hope this book sharpens your research axe.

INDEX